The Midnight Meal and Other Essays About Doctors, Patients, and Medicine

YALE UNIVERSITY PRESS/NEW HAVEN AND LONDON

The Midnight Meal

and Other Essays About Doctors, Patients, and Medicine

JEROME LOWENSTEIN, M.D.

Published with assistance from the Lucius
N. Littauer Foundation. Copyright ©
1997 by Yale University. All rights re-
served. This book may not be reproduced,
in whole or in part, including illustra-
tions, in any form (beyond that copying
permitted by Sections 107 and 108 of
the U.S. Copyright Law and except by
reviewers for the public press), without
written permission from the publishers.

Printed in the United States of America.

A catalogue record for this book is available from the British Library.

Library of Congress Cataloging-in
Publication Data
Lowenstein, Jerome.
The midnight meal and other essays
about doctors, patients, and medicine/
Jerome Lowenstein

p. cm.
Includes bibliographical references and
index.
ISBN 0-300-06816-6 (cloth: alk. paper)
1. Physician and patient. 2. Medicine–
Philosophy. 3. Physicians–Attitudes.
4. Interpersonal relations. I. Title.
[DNLM: 1. Physician-Patient Relations–
essays.2. Interprofessional Relations–
essays. 3. Philosophy, Medical–essays.
W9L917m 1996]   R727.3.L68 1997
610–dc20   DNLM/DC
for Library of Congress   96-26159
                                CIP

The paper in this book meets the guidelines for permanence and durability of
the Committee on Production Guidelines for Book Longevity of the Council
on Library Resources.

10 9 8 7 6 5 4 3 2 1

In memory of my parents, Fay and Sam,
and
for Ben, Lissa, Jon, Hannah, Lucy, Sylvie,
and my wife, Leahla

Not every patient can be saved, but his illness may be eased by the way the doctor responds to him—and in responding to him the doctor may save himself. But first he must become a student again; he must see that his silence and neutrality are unnatural. It may be necessary to give up some of his authority in exchange for his humanity, but as the old family doctors knew, this is not a bad bargain. In learning to talk to his patients, the doctor may talk himself back into loving his work. He has little to lose and everything to gain by letting the sick man into his heart. If he does, they can share, as few others can, the wonder, terror and exaltation of being on the edge of being.

Anatole Broyard, *Intoxicated by My Illness*

Contents

Contents

Preface

In these essays I speak to different listeners—to medical students, to
their teachers, to physicians whose lives and energies are committed to
the care of patients, and to patients themselves. The unifying theme is the
conviction that in sharing what Anatole Broyard termed "the wonder,
terror and exaltation of being on the edge of being" physicians will be
nourished and sustained. It is my belief that this will inevitably lead to
medical care that is more "humanistic" and compassionate. The origins
of many of the ideas, insights, and thoughts that appear in these essays can
be traced to my involvement with the program in Humanistic Medicine
that has been an integral part of the education of medical students and
house staff on the medical services at New York University Medical
Center for more than fifteen years. Weekly small group seminars on the
wards, in the Medical Intensive Care Unit, and in the AIDS Unit have
created a sanctioned portion of the curriculum which allows medical
students and young physicians to explore their responses to the process of
becoming physicians. The program in Humanistic Medicine has given
me the opportunity to work closely with an extraordinary group of

colleagues who serve as seminar leaders and to spend countless hours in small group discussions with medical students and young physicians-in-training.

Medical students and young physicians are more willing and able to examine and identify the feelings that underlie their daily interactions with patients than are many of my colleagues. We, physicians and medical educators, simply do not set aside the time to sit for an hour each week to explore our feelings and responses to our daily experiences. Most of us regard it as a luxury to "put a mark" on some comment or incident and examine it in greater depth with our colleagues. I strongly disagree. I have come to regard the opportunity to examine some of the many powerful experiences in my work with my colleagues as a necessity rather than a luxury. Howard Gardner, in *Creating Minds,* points out the importance of interactions with close colleagues in the process of creativity. These interactions in our seminars in Humanistic Medicine have led me to examine the process of becoming and remaining a caring physician and have been the stimulus to write this book.

Acknowledgments

It was with considerable trepidation that I presented my earliest plans to "teach humanistic medicine" to students and house staff to Dr. Saul J. Farber, chairman of the Department of Medicine and dean of the New York University School of Medicine. He has been a role model and teacher throughout my career. His lifelong commitment and selfless dedication to medical education have made him unique among the leaders in American medicine. I have heard him repeat lessons that he learned from his family and his teachers. Some of his teachings are so woven into my character that I can no longer recognize their origins. The qualities of humanism, which our program is intended to foster and nourish, are an integral part of the basic fabric of his life. He listened closely, questioned, and challenged as I outlined my still-embryonic plan, and in the end gave his full support to developing the Program in Humanistic Medicine.

A diverse and talented faculty has been drawn from the Wurzweiler School of Social Work of Yeshiva University, Hunter College, the Department of Psychiatry and the Primary Care Residency program at New York University Medical Center. Aaron Beckerman, ready to examine xiv and challenge any concept, was a "founding father" together with Charlie Rohrs, a very gifted, eclectic psychiatrist. Elsbeth Couch, a genius at hearing others' voices, along with Fred Wertzer and Ken Kahaner, who make it easy for others to find their voices, taught me to listen. Mack Lipkin, Jr., with his interest in teaching the skills of communication, brought to our program faculty members from the Primary Care program. Sarah Williams, Francesca Gany, Adina Kalet, Carol Mahon, and William Salazar added an important dimension to our program. Joshua Sherman, a lawyer, social worker, chaplaincy student, and author made his own unique contributions to our program when he was not at Oxford University.

The support of Dean David Scotch and Leslie Berlowitz and the Humanities Council of New York University were invaluable in initiating the program. After several years, I had the opportunity to meet with Bernard Schwartz, a member of the Board of Trustees of New York University School of Medicine, to describe our program. He felt strongly that what we were doing was very important and undertook to support the program as it expanded. He asked only that we come back to him and ask for more when we needed help. I will never forget our meeting which ended with a story about a "pushkie" (tzedakah box). During these years we have also received generous financial support from the Selma Terner Slater Fund, the Rose and Sherle Wagner Foundation, the Lucius Littauer Foundation, and the Conanima Foundation.

Laura Witt helped us in many ways in the beginning when we operated on a shoestring. Celia Harkin and Briedge McCarney have given much time to administrative and secretarial tasks. I am particularly fortunate that my secretary, Mildred Salwen, understood how I take care of patients and did everything to make it possible.

I am indebted to Kirk Jensen for encouraging me to write this book and for his thoughtful suggestions as it developed. Discussions with Margaret Mahoney at the Commonwealth Foundation and Sharon King at the Rockefeller Foundation finally convinced me to undertake this series of essays. I am deeply grateful to Richard Levin for his remarkably perceptive, imaginative, and valuable editorial suggestions, and to Jim

Dwyer for "entering into a dialogue" with this manuscript and for the xv
finely tuned suggestions that resulted. Several found their way into this
text. Special thanks go to my good friends Will Grossman, for his advice
as a cardiologist and critical reader, and Doris Battistella, for her gentle
editorial suggestions.

Dr. Lewis Thomas was the chairman of the Department of Medicine
when I began my training at Bellevue Hospital. He welcomed me to join
him in the exciting and rewarding life of academic medicine. Many years
later, he read my earliest essay and encouraged me to write this book. His
influence on my career has been very great; I owe him much.

The Midnight Meal

When I was a resident in medicine thirty-odd years ago, a regular feature of working through the evening in all teaching hospitals was the midnight meal for house staff. The midnight meal was a time to relax together with other house physicians, a time to unwind after a busy and stressful day. I am not aware of any formal study of the value these late evening communal meals had on the development of physicians, but I suspect that the late supper, which consisted simply of that day's leftovers, provided a fine opportunity to communicate with colleagues directly, rather than by beeper and phone, about many of the day's "medical leftovers." I remember midnight meals as a time when interns, residents, and, if they were fortunate, medical students assigned as clinical clerks spent an hour or so together, apart from their teachers and their patients. This was a time for getting help and information from colleagues who were further along in their training or who were simply more informed about a specific subject. They were also times for airing doubts, frustrations, or anger. There was a great deal of healthy laughter and a fair share of black humor.

Thirty years ago there were no intensive care units or coronary care 1

2   units. A few laboratory blood tests could be performed at night by the sole technician on duty, and emergency X-rays would be performed only if the need was clear to the night radiology technician. The environment in hospitals today is quite different. The pace is much more intense, and the evenings and nights are just as busy as the days. This has required changing the schedules for house staff. It is no longer reasonable to expect young physicians to work for forty-eight hours or more at a stretch. Elaborate schedules have been devised to accommodate the current expectations concerning medical care, particularly in tertiary care teaching hospitals. These have included limiting the length of periods on duty and creating night shifts and night float teams. Not surprisingly, the midnight meal is a thing of the past; it has been replaced by very concise "signouts" between day teams and night teams moving rapidly in opposite directions. Information passed from one "team" to the next is now limited to the most essential, usually technical, data. This is generally known as "passing the patient's numbers" (that is, laboratory results). I marvel at how effectively these signouts convey important information, but I know they cannot possibly fulfill all the functions that were served by the midnight meal. This late repast with its assorted leftovers achieved many of the ends for which we have had to create programs in humanistic medicine today.

This is not a call to go back in time. We have gained too much from sophisticated technology, and we have learned too much about the cellular and molecular aspects of disease, to return to the days of the general practitioner who made house visits carrying a small black bag, carefully recording the events of the patient's illness. While the experience of sitting in an elegant, intimate drawing room and listening to a Baroque concerto performed by the composer and fellow musicians on original instruments is not one we are likely to experience today, the critical component, the enjoyment of magnificent music performed in the company of friends, is clearly possible. The challenge is to identify and preserve, or recapture, the critical components of relationships in medicine—between colleagues and between physicians and patients—that we need to preserve. A good first step would be to devise some new equivalent of the midnight meal.

The Biomolecular Revolution

"It came like a lightning flash, like knowledge from the gods."[1] This was the reaction of biologist Edward Wilson to the report by James Watson and Francis Crick that established the structure of DNA and "broke the genetic code" in 1953. The Biomolecular Revolution that began with the breathtaking discoveries of Watson and Crick transformed science and medicine.[2] In the past forty years, the fields of molecular genetics, cell biology, and molecular biology have all come into being. An avalanche of new information and understanding has been associated in a "push-me, pull-me" fashion with dazzling technical advances. Medicine and medical education have not been the same since.

In 1983 Lewis Thomas wrote, "If I were a medical student or an intern, just getting ready to begin, . . . I would be apprehensive that my real job, caring for sick people, might soon be taken away, leaving me with the quite different occupation of looking after machines. I would be trying to figure out ways to keep this from happening."[3] Even as we marvel at the remarkable progress of medical science in the past forty years, it is not only medical students and those "getting ready to begin"

4   but also physicians and patients who share Lewis Thomas's concern. I also share his apprehension, but I am not worried that I, or my son in medical school, will be "looking after machines." The machines will look after themselves. I am much more concerned about the impact the Biomolecular Revolution has had and will continue to have on the relationship between students and their teachers, between physicians and their colleagues, and between physicians and their patients.

The effects of the Biomolecular Revolution on the structure of medicine have much in common with the effects of the Industrial Revolution on the structure of society. The Industrial Revolution, with the introduction of technologies for mass production, provided material goods to a great segment of society. However, the Industrial Revolution also led to the dissolution of the guilds, to the division of labor, and to the evolution of new social orders. The Industrial Revolution profoundly changed relationships among members of society. By analogy, the technology of the Biomolecular Revolution, which provides insights into the underlying biology of disease and makes truly effective treatments possible, may prove to have its greatest impact in medicine on the relationships that are important in our lives.

To understand the impact of the Biomolecular Revolution on relationships it is necessary to begin with the effects on medical education. Medical school curricula changed very little during the fifty years that followed the publication of the Flexner Report in 1910.[4] Preclinical studies—"basic science"—was traditionally subdivided into anatomy, microbiology, biochemistry, physiology, pharmacology, and pathology. The faculty responsible for teaching these subjects were few in number, mostly full-time members of the medical school faculty. They often conducted research, but unlike today, research grants were relatively easy to obtain and the pressure to publish was largely self-driven. The faculty's major commitments was to teaching and to providing support for the clinical services, for example, pathology, biochemistry, and bacteriology. Browse through old medical school yearbooks and you will find each of the preclinical departments represented by, at most, three or four faculty members, each of whom would likely be remembered vividly today by

their former students. The same faculty members who presented most of 5
the lectures also supervised the weekly laboratory sessions. These were
hours when students could clarify concepts, when a few students were
"turned on" to pursue a research project. This was a very important
experience; for some it was the beginning of a lifetime in investigative
medicine. I have vivid memories of many of the faculty who were my
teachers during those years. Faculty members were remembered by the
students because they influenced our early medical education and development. Some were very important role models; others were soon
forgotten.

The careful observations and the brilliant intuitive leap of Watson and
Crick established how the sequence of only four nucleotide bases in the
structure of DNA determined the information contained within the
gene. With dazzling speed, this discovery gave rise to the development of
techniques for isolating and characterizing fragments of genes, cloning
whole genes, inducing site-specific mutations, and inserting gene se-
quences into viruses or bacterial cells to direct the synthesis of biolog-
ically active products. Bioengineering was born. Almost overnight, the
status of research in medicine was elevated to a new level. Leaders emerging in this new field were identified, "cloned," and recruited to establish
divisions of molecular biology, cell biology, molecular genetics, and molecular pharmacology in preclinical departments of medical schools. The
influx of basic scientists and scientist-physicians transformed preclinical
departments of medical schools into what amounted in some instances to
research institutes, supported by the National Institutes of Health, housed
within the medical schools. This series of events contributed greatly to
the development and growth of the new fields of molecular and cell
biology, biophysics, and molecular genetics.

But these developments disturbed the ecology of medical education.
The responsibility for teaching medical students fell increasingly upon
young, full-time investigators in the basic sciences. Research, however,
was no longer the gentlemanly activity that full-time faculty engaged
in to enhance their knowledge as teachers. To allow enough time for
research and to reduce the burden on any one investigator, teaching

6   responsibilities were divided among a large group of young faculty. This brought medical students into contact with researchers who were often at the cutting edge of their fields and undoubtedly presented unique opportunities for those students with unusually receptive and fertile minds. But for many students this development resulted in the loss of contact with dedicated teachers in the preclinical sciences. It is not only the explosion of information in medicine that is responsible for the oft-heard complaint that what is taught in the preclinical years of medical school is "not relevant." The Biomolecular Revolution reduced the opportunities for close contact between students and faculty whose major commitment was to the education of medical students and weakened an important link that gave relevance to the preclinical sciences of biochemistry, physiology, and anatomy.

The experimental tools of medical research—mechanical transducers and recording kymographs, simple electrical recorders, and colorimeters, which had traditionally been used in laboratory exercises—were replaced by highly sophisticated equipment not suitable for large class use. Along with other factors such as time constraints, pressure from animal rights groups, and student dissatisfaction, this led to the virtual abandonment of laboratory exercises which represented a unique, often leisurely, opportunity for faculty and students to communicate. This was a serious loss. "Close student-faculty interaction" and "small-group learning," currently identified as the goals of curricular reform in many medical schools, were in fact the main focus of the laboratory exercises that have disappeared from the medical school curriculum for the preclinical years.

The Biomolecular Revolution has had equally dramatic and painful effects on teaching during the clinical years (usually the third and fourth years) of medical school. Historically, hospital wards were the classrooms in which medical students and young physicians learned clinical medicine. The word *clinical* comes from the Greek *kline,* meaning a bed. It was as true then as it is now that patients who require hospitalization suffer from illnesses that represent only a small and unrepresentative segment of clinical medicine. In the past, this limitation was seen as an acceptable trade-off balanced against the opportunity for students and young phy-

sicians to observe the evolution of illnesses from initial presentation,
through diagnosis and therapy, often to outcome. Patients usually remained in the hospital long enough for students to examine and re-
examine them, to learn much about disease, and to take the very important step of learning something about the person with the illness rather
than simply about the signs and symptoms of the disease. Today, as a result
of improved diagnostic techniques and shortened hospital stays, students
and house staff barely have time to learn the patient's name and diagnosis
before the patient is discharged.

Technology has improved diagnostic capabilities by many orders of
magnitude during the past two or three decades and has radically changed
the pattern of medical care in hospitals and the role of the teaching
hospital in medical education. As is the case with the new giant computers and linear accelerators in the physical sciences, the new diagnostic
instruments in medicine are so expensive that it is uneconomical (and
therefore unthinkable) that they be operated only during an eight-, ten-,
or even twelve-hour working day. As ancient gods were propitiated, these
machines must be used to justify their enormous cost. In other fields of
science, the introduction of such powerful and expensive instruments has
led to the development of teams of scientists who work in shifts throughout the day or to automation to permit the optimal utilization of these
"giant tools." Hospitals have more trouble adopting such a "no day no
night" strategy. The capacity to deal equally well with every level of
medical need at any hour of the day or night (and many modern hospitals
approach this standard) can represent the difference between life and
death for some patients. It does not follow that if the capacity exists to
perform a diagnostic or therapeutic procedure at any hour that the "giant
tools" must be utilized rather than be idle. Most patients do not benefit
from, or appreciate, being subjected to active care around-the-clock.
Rest has some distinct salutary role in the treatment of patients—even if
the diagnostic and therapeutic tools we employ are untiring!

Although the nursing profession has long operated on a shift system,
the medical profession had a tradition that valued, perhaps glorified, the
notion of the physician standing at the patient's bedside for the duration

8 of the crisis. This tradition paralleled the structure of physicians' responsibilities in teaching hospitals, which evolved in order to accommodate the dual responsibilities of patient care and teaching. Young physicians in training (interns and residents) provided around-the-clock coverage, spending periods as long as 48 to 60 hours on duty and frequently working 100 hours per week in the hospital. Teaching rounds were made on a daily basis, usually in the morning, by attending physicians. Though the on-duty hours were long, the rhythm of most services in hospitals dictated that evenings and nights were generally quiet except for medical emergencies.

Today medical care is a twenty-four-hour affair. The clinical chemistry laboratories and the X-ray department operate around-the-clock, it is possible to have the most sophisticated radiologic procedure at any hour, and treatment does not await the dawn. Lives are saved by this around-the-clock care. However, the intensity of care in hospitals created a great strain on the young physicians who were on duty for long periods. Concern about sleep deprivation and fatigue culminated, in New York State, in the promulgation of a series of regulations limiting working hours for house staff. Most hospitals were not able to recruit additional house staff since the pool of medical school graduates was limited and funding was tight. Reducing the working hours meant that fewer house-staff physicians would be on duty at any given time. This change came about at the same time that reimbursement plans were mandating shorter hospital stays and more rapid turnover of patients. As a consequence, although the working day was shorter, it was more intense. The physical, intellectual, and emotional demands on house staff increased as the working hours decreased.

The recently graduated physicians who had experienced the stress of round-the-clock, high intensity care heralded these changes in work schedules as welcome and important reforms. Some older physicians and clinical faculty of medical schools bemoaned the fact that "the days of the giants had passed." In fact, despite the very long hours, those days of golden memory were, I believe, far less intense and stressful than those experienced by house staff today. In my judgment, it was crucial that

work schedules be changed in response to round-the-clock intensive care 9
in hospitals, but these changes were accomplished at a very great price.

The most serious consequences of the Biomolecular Revolution can
be seen in the profound effects on the relationship between young physicians and their patients. Shortened hospital stays and rapid turnover virtually dictate that those aspects of medical care, diagnostic as well as therapeutic, that do not require the technology of the hospital be performed
in the outpatient setting. The current hospital reimbursement system,
which categorizes all illnesses into diagnosis-related groups (DRGs), encourages the practice of viewing patients as "examples of disease." While
this form of reductionism may be sound from the point of view of medical economics, it does not provide a sound introduction to the process of
becoming a physician. I am certain that it has a subtle or subliminal effect
on how physicians think about individual patients. Learning about illness
as opposed to disease—that is, the ways in which patients' lives are affected
by disease and the very great variety of individual responses to disease—is
low on the list of priorities during a busy day in a busy week for most
physicians-in-training. I rarely meet an intern or resident who does not
place greater importance on knowing a patient's blood count than on
knowing the basic details of the patient's life. The blood count is sometimes more important in the totality of a patient's medical care than
whether the patient has a family, a home, or a job, but I doubt that this is
usually the case.

The increasing complexity of modern diagnostic procedures and
treatments and time constraints are held responsible for the need to determine priorities in patient care. Lewis Thomas stated it very simply: "The
new medicine works. It is a vastly more complicated profession, with
more things to be done on short notice on which issues of life and death
depend. . . . If I develop the signs and symptoms of malignant hypertension, or cancer of the colon, or subacute bacterial endocarditis, I want as
much comfort and friendship as I can find at hand, but mostly I want to
be treated quickly and effectively so as to survive, if that is possible."[5]

To my mind, this "new medicine" is no less dependent on the
physician-patient relationship than medicine was before the Biomolecu-

10   lar Revolution. Medicine has always involved the physician and the patient in an intense, complex, and important relationship. For the patient,
the effects and consequences of illness are far greater than the sum of the
cellular and molecular events that define the disease. To understand illness and to intervene effectively, physicians need to grasp some of the
patient's narrative, to understand the context of meanings in which the
disease is at work. The more serious and life-threatening the illness,
the greater is the need of the patient to experience the patient-physician
relationship in its broadest original sense. Stripped of the relationship
between the physician and the patient, medical care, however scien-
tifically based, technically refined, and accurate, can be a frightening
affair. Despite our increasing acceptance of technology, we all feel a need
for some human connection. Few of us would be comfortable having
surgery performed by the best programmed robot. Although the technical support for astronauts in space is awesome in its sophistication, I
strongly suspect that the voice of their colleagues at Mission Control
plays an equally important role in the emotional support of these space
technicians.

It is not only the patient who stands to suffer as the traditional patient-
physician relationship is lost. From its origins, the relationship between
physicians (read "shamans," "healers," "medicine men") and patients has
represented more to both parties than simply the delivery of health care.
The doctor-patient interaction took place when life and death hung in a
precarious balance; it is not surprising that it should have had a powerful
emotional effect on both parties. The helplessness, uncertainty, and fear
experienced by patients evoke resonant emotions in the physician. The
physician and the patient have always shared these highly charged emotional experiences. Aristotle recognized the salutary emotional response
to such experiences. The term *catharsis* refers to the feeling of "being
more alive," "invigorated," or "in touch" when we experience intense
emotions. These intense emotional interactions should be as much a part
of the relationship between patients and physicians in today's highly sophisticated, technologically advanced, biomolecular era as they were
when the therapeutic armamentarium of the doctor was limited to

leeches, purges, and nostrums. But few physicians today, and probably even fewer patients, would use such terms in describing their medical experiences or physician-patient encounters. Physicians who are more intensely engaged in these interactions experience a sense of fulfillment or even exhilaration in response to the intense engagement with their own and their patients' deepest emotions. The writings of William Carlos Williams, Richard Seltzer, and others portray physicians practicing around the turn of the century, long before the Biomolecular Revolution, as "better nourished." The suffering and grief experienced by the patient and family were more readily absorbed and shared by the physician in the setting of the patient's home than in today's modern hospital where death is usually seen as a defeat. Death in the home seems to draw people together in their loss. House calls, though hardly a cost-effective form of medical encounter today, served an important function. This setting allowed the physician a glimpse of the patient's world. In the home, the patient could be validated. "Although you see me now as weak, failing, vulnerable, look at these signs that show that I was strong, young, accomplished, not alone." I have heard the same experiences described by colleagues who still visit some of their very ill or dying patients in their homes.

The legacy of the Biomolecular Revolution will be a new medicine in which the fundamental biology of many diseases will come to be known on a cellular and molecular level. These insights will translate into the cure of diseases that have eluded treatment throughout our history. It is hard for me to imagine any aspect of our lives in which the prospects for the future are as exciting and promising. However, we will have to find, or rediscover, ways to sustain and nurture important relationships in medicine—between students and teachers, between colleagues, and between patients and physicians—if we are to avoid painful losses as medicine is transformed by the Biomolecular Revolution.

Can You Teach Compassion?

That which comes from the heart, goes to the heart
—*Moshe Ibn Ezra,* Shirat Yisrael *(Songs of Israel), eleventh century*

The question has often been put to me, Do you really think you can teach compassion? This question cannot be answered briefly; it calls for a rather lengthy response. First, the term *compassion* can be taken as a form of shorthand, the equivalent of an acronym, for the many qualities that define humanistic attitudes and behavior in medicine. Compassion also stands for empathy, respect, a recognition of the uniqueness of another individual, and the willingness to enter into a relationship in which not only the knowledge but the intuitions, strengths, and emotions of both the patient and the physician can be fully engaged. Is compassion a skill? Can compassion or any of the other qualities mentioned be taught? If teaching is taken to mean instructing and providing clear protocols, lists, and methods, the answer would clearly be no. But this is certainly teaching in the most restricted sense. No doubt a body of information and a theoretical framework exist that address the process of professional devel-

opment—including the development of attitudes and patterns of behavior, even compassion—and that would be termed humanistic. It has
always seemed to me that this theoretical framework is more valuable in
our attempts to understand the process of professional growth than in our
efforts to bring it about. The question is not whether there is a body of
information to be learned but whether it can be taught.

There is a paradox in teaching medicine. On the one hand, given the
rapid developments in the neurosciences, genetics, and cell and molecular biology, students and young physicians know a great deal more than
their teachers about the basic science underlying the understanding and
treatment of disease. On the other hand, it is quite evident that the
experience of having practiced medicine, which sets the teacher ahead of
the students in many ways, is not readily taught. Given these limitations,
teachers in medicine can only hope to facilitate the development of
students or young physicians, challenging and stimulating them and acting as role models. Viewed in this way, teaching compassion and teaching
medicine have much in common. There is at least one important difference, however. Students do not enter medical school with an "embryonic
knowledge" of electrocardiography or a "strong sense" of acid-base physiology, but many of the qualities that we associate with compassion are
already clearly evident in the earliest contact between medical students
and patients. While electrocardiography and acid-base physiology must
be learned, de novo, compassion, empathy, and sensitivity are qualities
that can develop early in life and that reflect cultural, family, social, and
uniquely personal experiences. When does this development cease? Are
the attitudes and behaviors of the young women and men who are entering medical school or who are at the start of their clinical training, already
determined?

In one of our Humanistic Medicine seminars,[1] the small group of
medical students, interns, and residents was challenged to respond to the
question, Do you think we can teach you compassion? After an uncom-
fortably long pause, an intern said in a voice that seemed to convey both
anger and shame, "I don't know if you can teach compassion, but you
surely can teach the opposite!" He was referring to a phenomenon that is

14   well known in the development of medical students and house staff. At a
minimum, it might be termed "hardening," a *learned* insensitivity to the
pain and suffering and the needs of patients. At its worst it is seen as a
dehumanization of patients who are referred to, in order of decreasing
humanity, as "MIs," "hits," "crocks," "gomers," and "shpozes."[2] This
process, which Robert Jay Lifton has described as "psychic numbing,"
occurs with remarkable speed, often within the first one or two years of
clinical training.[3] The regularity with which this desensitization occurs
challenges the notion, which I have often heard expressed, that one
cannot change the behavior and attitudes of young men and women
already in their middle twenties.

The question is not whether we *can* teach compassion but rather
whether we will teach compassion or its opposite. I have heard students
being taught the opposite of compassion. Some house staff caution naive
medical students against "becoming too involved" with certain patients
or counsel that "time spent with the books" will get them further than
learning more about any single patient. Academic success and recognition seem to go to the stronger and faster. Early in their training, medical
students are troubled by the realization that many of the angry and embit-
tered physicians they see as house staff or attending physicians on the
hospital wards stood in their places only a few years earlier.

Why are we faced, at this time, with these questions about teaching
compassion? Compassion, empathy, respect for the uniqueness of others
are behaviors and values that have always been regarded as the very qualities that lead young men and women to enter the field of medicine. They
were never taught, as such, but rather were nurtured and reinforced by
prolonged contact with teachers who served as role models and with
patients. As the pace of medicine has accelerated in the second half of
the twentieth century, the slow educational process by which physicians
"learned compassion" suffered. Physicians today, in their roles as teachers,
complain that they feel overburdened by their responsibilities for the care
of patients whose illnesses are complex and often require the expertise of
teams of specialists. Many physicians are intimidated by the very large
body of knowledge they must master and transmit to students and house

officers. One way of coping with these very understandable feelings is to narrow one's focus, to deal with only that part of the disease one knows best and leave the rest to others with different areas of expertise. This does not work well in the care of patients, nor does it make for good teaching and role modeling. To focus on a specific problem, no matter how important or interesting, it is usually necessary to direct attention away from the patient, where all problems intersect.

If it be granted that it is possible and necessary to teach compassion, where is the time and where is the place? My response is a personal and perhaps idiosyncratic one. It requires some explanation. For many years I have taken pride in my ability to teach students and house staff. I try to approach clinical problems from the point of understanding the underlying pathophysiology; I feel that pathophysiology provides a solid underpinning for differential diagnosis, provides a sound direction for treatment, and is instructive for students and house staff. In recent years, on a busy teaching service, I found little time to explore with students or house staff issues related to the lives of patients that were presented to me on daily rounds. Patients' understanding of their illnesses or their responses rarely found a place in my daily teaching rounds. Was this because I felt these issues were unimportant or unrelated to the care of patients? Certainly not. I felt that I was coping as well as I could with the time pressures of teaching on an active medical service. Looking back on this time, however, I now recognize that another subliminal factor was responsible for my ordering of priorities. I recall that, as a student and house officer, my role models among attending physicians were familiar with all the recent medical literature; they challenged us to understand complex pathophysiology. The attending physicians whom I and my peers tried to avoid, if any excuse could be found, tended to fill our teaching sessions or rounds with anecdotes and platitudes about patients. I will never be able to accurately reconstruct what they were trying to teach, but I realize now that when I became an attending physician I felt a deep discomfort, during my rounds, whenever I heard myself deviating from the image of one of my rigorous scientific role models.

I was keenly aware that an important element of medical education

16   was not being addressed, by me or by many of my colleagues. I found myself quite comfortable discussing with students and house staff their experiences and responses to patients as well as my own observations, feelings, pleasures, and discomforts in physician-patient interactions in our weekly Humanistic Medicine small-group meetings with medical students and house staff. Yet despite my involvement in the Humanistic Medicine Program, it was rare that I would raise one of these issues on daily morning rounds. I restricted these discussions to our afternoon small-group meetings, although the meetings were with the same group of students and house staff! Two or three years ago, as an experiment, I decided to integrate my "afternoon" style into my morning attending rounds. This was not exactly a planned or deliberate step. I found myself increasingly uncomfortable with the manner in which our students and house staff glossed over critical information in their daily morning case presentations. Patients were described, in a word, as "homeless," "un-domiciled," "an IVDA," or "a shooter." The traditional presentation of the patient's social history was frequently no more than a recitation of how much the patient smoked and whether the patient used drugs or alcohol and in which form. The most streamlined case presentations boiled this information down to a simple formula, "x pack-years, y bags, and z quarts daily." I remember vividly the first morning when I interrupted an intern in the middle of his opening sentence, "This is the first hospital admission of this thirty-five-year-old IVDA . . ." I asked, "Would our thinking or care be different if you began your history by telling us that this is a thirty-five-year-old Marine veteran who has been addicted to drugs since he served, with valor, in Vietnam?" There was an embarrassed hush. As I left the ward later that morning, I reflected that the few minutes taken up by my question might have been my most important contribution of the day, possibly more instructive than my comments about pneumocystis pneumonia, arterial oxygen saturation, and respiratory alkalosis. I have continued to insist that patients be "personalized" in case presentations and find that I have been able to integrate details about patients' perceptions, responses, and needs without sacrificing attention to other aspects of clinical medicine. I am no less rigorous in my analysis

of clinical data, nor has my interest in pathophysiology waned. The
response of students and house staff reassure me that I have not crossed
over to "anecdotes and platitudes." I have come to believe that the time
and place to teach compassion are the time and place in which all of the
rest of medicine is taught.

If we are to preserve and nourish humanistic values in medicine, if we
are to teach compassion, it would seem to me that the process must begin
with a clear recognition that this is the responsibility of the faculty who
teach medical students and young physicians. It would be tragic if humanistic medicine were to become "alternative medicine" or a subject—
worse yet, an elective subject—in the curriculum. The presentation of
courses on the history of medicine and on humanism in literature has
provided a forum for emphasizing the importance of the patient's narrative and for examining characters presented by Thomas Mann, Lev Tol-
stoy, and Aleksandr Solzhenitsyn, patients described by Oliver Sachs, and
the ways in which illness transforms people's lives. These courses engage
ethicists, sociologists, and talented educators from other fields in teaching
medicine, but the presentation of such important concepts as "small
museum pieces," to my mind, falls short of the real need in medicine
today. If "teaching compassion" is a part of teaching medicine, it should
be the responsibility of all those who teach clinical medicine.[4] I am sure
that there are faculty who would reject the notion that "teaching compassion" is their responsibility. I would view them in the same way I view
a teacher of medicine who rejects the idea of teaching physical diagnosis
or pathophysiology. This person might be a gifted and valuable teacher,
but this outlook is a distinct limitation. As Hashim Khan, a legendary
squash player and teacher wrote, "I once knew a man who played the
piano with gloves. He played well, for a man with gloves on."[5]

Changing physicians' attitudes is not an easy task. When I feel pessi-
mistic about the possibility of teaching compassion, I am reassured by the
realization that our society has become very adept at and indeed dependent on its capacity to change attitudes and behaviors. How else can we
interpret the rapid changes we see in such matters as fashion, in clothing,
in diet, or the craze for jogging? These are not random or chance events.

18   The remarkable changes in diet, cigarette smoking, and exercise in the United States in response to a well-planned education program initiated by the National Heart and Lung Institute and the American Heart Association are clear evidence that behavior patterns, food preferences, and life styles, though deeply ingrained, are subject to change. It seems to me that the motivation for such changes in behavior and attitudes derives from promised rewards—prevention of heart attacks or strokes, an enhanced feeling of well-being or physical attractiveness.

What then are the promised rewards for medical students, house staff, and physicians who enter more fully into relationships that are time-consuming, painful, and demanding? And how are the energies of the teachers to be renewed? I suppose the answer for each of us will be different. For some, experiencing the richness of the relationship may be sufficient reward, but for many this will not suffice. I believe that it should be possible to demonstrate that physicians' behavior, and by this I mean to imply "humanistic" attitudes and relationships, correlate with "rewards" such as physician satisfaction, patient satisfaction, better compliance with therapy, and less conflict regarding therapeutic decisions or malpractice issues. The medical community expects physicians to change long-held attitudes and patterns of behavior in response to the findings of research describing new forms of treatment or diagnostic tests. Careful and verifiable studies of the physician-patient interaction could affect physician attitudes toward the value of teaching compassion.

I recognize that the nurturing of humanistic qualities for which I am making a plea cannot be achieved by a chance remark on rounds or even by role modeling, but requires a dedicated self-conscious effort. That dedicated effort need not be a formal didactic conference; in fact, as we have found, may be better organized as an unstructured block of time set aside simply to "look at" some event that has taken place or to explore the feelings related to some interaction. There is little doubt in my mind that our weekly Humanistic Medicine sessions have contributed significantly to my growth as a physician and a teacher. These encounters have given me valuable insights into the struggles of students and house staff to maintain their sense of compassion and connectedness to patients. Some of the issues they face are familiar. I recall similar struggles, and I face some of the same issues today. Other concerns are unique; at times I find myself shocked, angered, or depressed, but at other times I am greatly buoyed by the idealism and courage of these young men and women. I have come to recognize that just as there are students who are very adept at grappling with complex issues of differential diagnosis or pathophysiology, there are also students who display unusual qualities of understanding and sensitivity in their interactions with patients. Some of these students have themselves faced serious illness or dealt with loss or geographic dislocation, and these experiences have left them better prepared to help their patients than are the older experienced physicians who are their teachers. These strengths of students should be recognized and rewarded when we evaluate academic excellence. Similarly, the strengths of the faculty in teaching compassion should be recognized and rewarded in the academic setting.

Finally, my experiences in teaching compassion have lead me to respond to the rhetorical question posed earlier, How are the energies of the teachers renewed? Just as I feel the physician-patient relationship provides moments of intense gratification and "connexion"[6] that are important in nurturing the physician, I believe that "teaching compassion" has given my relationship with students and house staff an added element of excitement, pleasure, and renewal for me as a teacher.

Coughs, Clouds, and Ice

The importance of precision in language is evident in the more than twenty different terms Inuits use to describe ice and in the great many types of clouds distinguished by Native Americans.[1] These distinctions are drawn because they serve a purpose. They are necessary in deciding when to plant or harvest, when to travel, when to set out on a hunt. In medicine an equally precise vocabulary of descriptive terms was once employed. The racking cough of the patient with active tuberculosis, the weak, ineffectual hacking cough of the chronic bronchitic, the "whoop" and the "croup" were as carefully defined, and carried the same practical significance, as the names given to clouds and ice. I am not certain whether meteorologic data and satellite weather forecasting have supplanted the descriptions of clouds and ice. It does seem clear that the chest X-ray and the chest CT scan have supplanted the careful distinctions among different patterns of cough and the colorful descriptions of breath sounds and noises in the chest. The rich descriptive lexicon that once characterized medical writing has been replaced by a stylized, stereotyped jargon that relies heavily on abbreviations, acronyms, neologisms, and pseudo-quantitation ("four out of ten chest pain"). Most medical students and house staff don't see much value in the precise description, or perhaps even in the detection, of a heart murmur given present diagnostic techniques, which allow a viewer to see each of the chambers and valves of the heart and observe blood flow in vivid, if not living, color.

What has been lost by the introduction of this extraordinary technology? I suspect that for the Native American and the Inuit, replacing the age-old descriptions of clouds and ice by scientific data, even granting for the moment that the information is more accurate, must reflect a painful loss of continuity with a tradition and with a physical place—the land. Language plays an important role in maintaining a tradition. When a generation of children acquires a new language, whether as a result of assimilation into a new culture or as a consequence of the evolution of the language itself, a painful gap is created in that society. Equally, in societies or cultures in which the land or the sea plays a central role in the belief system, as it does for Native Americans, Inuits, or sailors, the loss of firsthand experience with the environment must create a very real sense of isolation. Sociologists have recognized and written much about the disruptive effects of technological advances on these societies. It seems to me that there may be some merit to looking at technological advances in medicine, viewed as a society, to answer the question, What is lost? There is no question that medicine has gained remarkable diagnostic capabilities that can readily be translated into the relief of suffering, prolongation of life, and very likely, depending on how you add up the totals, great economic savings. Just as the loss of the firsthand experience of clouds and ice can be a painful and disruptive experience for societies closely involved with their physical place, the new technology and the change in the language of medicine have led to a disturbing separation of the physician from the "physical land of medicine," that is, from the patient and the physical body. Medicine, at its best, requires the physician to feel about and to regard the patient in much the same manner in which aboriginal peoples regard the land, as something sensate, special, even holy. For all the remarkable and dramatic benefits that have come about from the new

22   diagnostic tools and the new understanding of the cellular and molecular basis of disease, there has clearly been a loss of this sense of direct contact which, it seems to me, is critical for the sustenance of both the physician and patient.

The language of medicine today is clearly different from that of fifty or even twenty-five years ago. These changes in the language of medicine have strained its traditions. Would it have been possible to replace the rich and multilayered discourse of the midnight meals with the shorthand alphabet soup of letters and numbers used in today's signouts, if the language of medicine had not already changed? The transformation of language cuts off all but the most pragmatic and immediate communication between students of medicine and their teachers or mentors. In addition, it affects the process of role modeling, which is a critical part of the physician's development. I suspect that the change in language and the closely related shifts in paradigms also contribute significantly to the increasingly apparent gap between physicians and patients. The call for the "old-time physician" is not a call for a wise old man with a little black bag and a few harmless (and useless) nostrums, but a yearning for communication in a common language. Importantly that common language included a great number of terms for hope, reassurance, strength, and courage.

Treating Chronic Illness

When I was a medical student, internists were referred to as "diagnosticians." This term carried the image of a very knowledgeable physician, skilled in interpreting subtle findings in order to arrive at a difficult, or at times brilliant, diagnosis. The term *internist,* a specialist in internal medicine, identified an intellectual elite in medicine; internal medicine attracted many of the brightest students in every medical school class. Things have changed. Today, medical students see internists as dissatisfied physicians, undervalued, beleaguered by endless paperwork, overburdened with the care of patients with chronic illness or functioning as "gatekeepers" in managed care systems.

What changed in the past thirty years? Until the middle of this century, most medical care was in the hands of general practitioners, whose training was limited to the completion of an internship. Most of the care provided by family doctors or general practitioners involved the treatment of acute illnesses, which were frequently self-limited. Spontaneous recovery was common, and some treatments helped; but occasionally the acute disease was fatal. Pneumonia and other infections were treated with

24   antibiotics, but the choice of antibiotics was limited. Cardiac failure and some cardiac arrhythmias called for treatment with digitalis or digoxin, quinidine, and at times, intravenous mercurial diuretics. Asthma, when severe, was treated with subcutaneous epinephrine. There were no effective medical treatments for chronic illnesses such as emphysema, hypertension, rheumatoid arthritis, peptic ulcer, colitis, cancer, depression, or schizophrenia. The few diseases for which long-term treatment was commonly prescribed, such as tuberculosis and rheumatic fever, were treated in sanatoria or special convalescent facilities. Routine examinations, such as yearly checkups, and preventive medicine, except for immunization, were virtually unknown. General practitioners knew their patients through repeated contacts related to acute illness in one or another member of the family. Patients were referred to internists when the diagnosis was unclear or when an unusual disease was suspected. Internists were "diagnosticians" by virtue of their advanced training and their access to hospitals that housed diagnostic facilities such as X-ray departments, chemistry and microbiology laboratories, and pathology laboratories. Diagnosticians devoted most of their time to consultation either in the office or in the hospital, and many were renowned for their abilities as teachers in medical schools.

The development of bronchodilator drugs, antihypertensive agents, corticosteroids, and nonsteroidal anti-inflammatory drugs, inhibitors of gastric acid secretion, cytotoxic drugs, antidepressant and psychotropic agents—all within the past thirty or forty years—have radically transformed the way medicine is practiced. These new therapeutic agents have made it possible to treat and to control the symptoms or modify the outcome of many chronic illnesses but, with few exceptions, do not *cure* the diseases for which they are prescribed. The ability to treat these common chronic diseases has had profound and far-reaching consequences. It has been said, usually critically, that "more surgeons mean more surgery." It appears equally true that more *treatments* mean more treatment of chronic illness. In the debate about the increasing costs of health care, too little attention has been paid to the fact that more illnesses are now treatable. Willard Gaylin wrote, "The greatest part of the increase in health care

costs can best be understood as a result not of the failure of medicine but   25
of its successes."[1] It seems likely that this trend to more treatment (and
higher health care costs) will accelerate in the next decade or two as
medical knowledge and technology devise new and better treatments,
but not necessarily cures, for chronic diseases such as cancer, degenerative
joint disease, atherosclerotic cardiac and cerebrovascular disease, congestive heart failure, AIDS, and Alzheimer's disease.

As patients with chronic illness live longer, requiring treatment with
powerful new drugs that have potentially life-threatening side effects, it is
not surprising that the treatment of chronic illness has become increasingly the responsibility of internists who have more expertise in treating
specific diseases and greater experience in the use of these drugs. Paradoxically, while internists have taken on more of the responsibility for
treating chronic illness, family doctors and general practitioners are now
able to undertake complex diagnostic evaluations through direct access to
facilities that offer advanced radiologic and other imaging studies and, in
effect, provide consultation by highly trained and skilled radiologists,
pathologists, microbiologists, immunologists, and biochemists. Any physician can send specimens to commercial laboratories which offer a range
of diagnostic studies far exceeding the capacity of the finest hospital
laboratory. The turnabout in roles is nearly complete. General practitioners and family physicians are now the "diagnosticians"; they refer the
patient to a specialist—a general internist or internist with subspecialty
training—for management and chronic care! With few exceptions, internists and medical subspecialists devote most of their practice to the care of
chronic illness. Even physicians trained in infectious diseases, long considered a specialty in which dramatic benefits could be gained after short-
term treatment, now find themselves treating patients with diseases such
as AIDS which, with current therapy, is evolving into a treatable, though
incurable, chronic illness.

The rapidity with which these changes in patterns of practice have
come about may be responsible for what appears to be a disruption in
well-established patterns by which young physicians learn to care for
patients. Traditionally medical education was hospital-based and focused

26 largely on the diagnosis, pathophysiology, and short-term management of acute illness, or acute exacerbations of chronic illness. These were the areas of expertise of the specialists, the diagnosticians, who were the attending physicians and teachers of medical students and house officers. The shift in the focus of internal medicine from diagnosis to the treatment of chronic illness has raised major issues regarding where medicine should be taught, what ought to be taught, and by whom. These are not questions raised solely by medical educators or health care planners. Students and physicians in training sense that the medicine they learn in the hospital is quite different from the real world of clinical practice. Training programs, hospital-based and focused on acute illness, are criticized as "irrelevant" to the needs of physicians who contemplate a career in general medicine. This criticism has become a rallying point for groups who would place more emphasis on family care, primary care, ambulatory care, holistic care, and alternative medicine. For me, the designation "irrelevant" seems grossly overstated.

The majority of medical students and house staff seem to recognize that the core of primary care or internal medicine today is the treatment of chronic illness. For some students this seems an attractive feature, while for others it appears to be a significant deterrent to choosing internal medicine as a career. A new class of internist-specialists has evolved, physicians who practice largely in hospitals, perform consultations and procedures such as endoscopy, bronchoscopy, renal dialysis, or invasive cardiac procedures, but devote little time to chronic care. The lifestyle of these physicians is not very different from the earlier model of the diagnostician as a consultant concerned with diagnosis, pathophysiology, and acute short-term treatment.

The evolution of medical care from acute care to the care and treatment of chronic illness represents a very great challenge to medical education and to physicians. The devotion of more time to ambulatory care in house staff training programs is an appropriate response but does not fully address the problem. Preparing physicians to care for people with chronic illness must start early in medical school. What does this involve?

What are the critical components of caring for someone with chronic illness? First, an appreciation of the natural history of disease plays a critical role. This aspect is often neglected in teaching medical students and house officers because the training programs traditionally focus on the presenting signs and symptoms, the various tests required to establish a diagnosis, the pathophysiology, and the treatment of acute illnesses. The course and outcome of chronic illnesses, the likelihood of stroke or heart attack in hypertension, renal failure in diabetes mellitus, the disease-free interval after cancer chemotherapy, or the asymptomatic period following HIV infection are addressed largely in terms of statistics and probabilities. Textbooks of medicine have little to say about what transpires between the diagnosis and the outcome, during the years the patient is being treated for these chronic diseases. This is a body of information that the best doctors acquire by carefully observing many patients and closely following the course of their illnesses. This always necessitates a deep understanding of the underlying pathophysiology of the disease. How else can one understand the factors that might accelerate or delay the progression of patients with chronic renal disease to end-stage renal failure and uremia, how else can the physician intelligently treat the patient with chronic congestive heart failure and reduced myocardial function, or effectively support the patient with cognitive impairment and slowly progressive dementia? At its best, the treatment of chronic illness focuses not only on the common features of the disease but on the wide range of differences in the way the disease progresses or remits and on the subtle variations in the manifestations of the disease.

Knowledge of the natural history of the disease is as important as a knowledge of the pharmacology of the medications in evaluating whether a patient's symptoms represent progression of the disease or an adverse drug reaction. This necessitates close listening to the patient whose illness is the manifestation of the disease. This is not an exercise in detective work, trying to dissect the underlying disease from the patient's complaints. In many ways the seemingly idiosyncratic aspects of the patient's response to a disease are, in fact, as much features of the illness as

28 are the characteristic physical findings, biochemical changes, or radiographic signs, that is, they are inseparable. Understanding disease and the many ways it is manifested as illness enables the physician to care for the patient in a unique manner. Each patient contributes measurably to the education of the physician. The capacity to learn about disease from a careful study of patients' illnesses is one of the distinguishing characteristics of those physicians whom I have come to respect as teachers and role models and of those doctors whom I search out as a physician for myself, my family, my friends, and my patients.

There is another aspect to caring for patients with chronic illness. I have consciously avoided the term *chronically ill,* which for me conjures up the image of a patient with a never-ending succession of complaints, new symptoms, recurrent ailments, and total involvement with illness. Though this is the sad and terrible plight of some patients, for many chronic illness is only a part of life, sharing a place with their interests, habits, loves, aspirations, accomplishments, and other burdens which, at times, dwarf their chronic illness. The best care of patients with chronic illness engages the physician and the patient in a relationship in which the full range of the strengths and knowledge of each play an important role. For the patient, this relationship shares with other support systems, family or close friends, a critical role in determining the impact, and outcome, of the illness on the patient's life. Studies of patients with a wide range of diseases have found that the outcome in chronic diseases is greatly affected by many factors which appear to relate more to the patient's life history, education, family supports, and emotional well-being than to the conventional indices of disease severity or to the therapies employed.[2]

For the physician, the relationship that evolves during the care of chronic illness carries with it the potential for a unique emotional reward, one that resonates with the undertones of "healing." Healing not in the sense of "making well," "curing" or "saving a life" but that process which in some way responds to the pain or loss incurred by illness and helps alleviate or lessen its effects. Many internists today accept and derive deep satisfaction from the shift in their role from "diagnostician" to a physician dedicated to the care of patients with chronic illness. They have learned

from their experience and from their patients, far more than from textbooks, what is needed to assume this new role. The field of internal
medicine cannot afford to assume that the next generation of medical
students and young physicians will acquire this knowledge in the same
slow, experiential manner.

Patients as Teachers

Saul was a journalist and writer.[1] I had been introduced to him a few years earlier and knew several of his close friends. When I learned that he had been admitted to University Hospital, I felt that I should stop in to visit him. I knew that the visit would be difficult, one that I did not look forward to. How do you make small talk with a vigorous, productive forty-five-year-old man who has just been told that he has leukemia? I proceeded with considerable trepidation, but without a plan. As I entered his room, a private room on the medical floor, I had the impression that he and his wife had just arrived. They looked out of place and bewildered. I introduced myself, mentioning several of our common friends. Formalities and small talk were quickly put aside, perhaps because of our mutual awareness of the seriousness of his situation. What do I say now? Something seemed to push me to go beyond a simple, "If I can be of any help . . ." Instead I found myself offering advice about how Saul might prepare himself for the difficult weeks and months ahead. I explained that he need not exchange his jogging suit for pajamas or a hospital gown. There was nothing to stop him from filling the room with photographs of

his family, books, and a CD player so that he could hear music throughout the day. I could not recall ever giving that sort of advice to a patient
before. Thinking about it, I chalked it up to my own discomfort. Perhaps
this was an idea about dealing with frightening illness that I had formulated but never clearly articulated before. As I left the room, I remarked
that I would visit with Saul again the next day. When I returned there
were signs that Saul had "moved in." Family photographs, books, and a
small refrigerator lined one wall. He greeted me, with a broad smile, in
his running suit. He asked me to sit down and began to relate the events
of the past week, from noting "small bruises" over his legs, to his visit to a
local physician, the discovery of the abnormal white blood cell count and
the news that he had leukemia. This was not a recitation of the series of
steps that had brought him to this terrible point, which is the way I might
have characterized the sequence, but was intended to be a background
briefing for the many questions he had prepared for me concerning his
disease and the treatments he would be undergoing. I explained that I did
not feel qualified or knowledgeable enough to answer many of his questions; he was under the care of a fine hematologist. He was not easily
deterred. A lifetime as a journalist and his skills as an interviewer became
evident as he led me into a discussion of many difficult aspects of illness.
Part of his remarkable response to this illness and hospitalization was his
ability to "interview" each person who walked into his room. During the
course of his long illness, countless attending physicians, nurses, aides,
phlebotomy technicians, residents, interns, and medical students came
into his room, whether to perform some small task or to deliver much
awaited results of the most recent blood count or bone marrow examinations. He knew them all by name, knew something about their lives, and
knew, through his own close observation, whom he could trust to give an
honest answer or attend to some need, and whom to call when he needed
reassurance. Over time I began to recognize that his lifelong orientation
as an inquiring and trained observer provided him with a remarkably
effective means of coping. The many physicians, students, nurses, aides,
and technicians involved in his care came to know him as an individual
not as "the man who needs platelets and a fever work up." He managed to

32   retain his identity through some very difficult times. When he lost his hair as result of chemotherapy, he wore a baseball cap and when his mouth was so sore that he could not smile or speak, he listened and gestured. Most striking was his ability to ask for information, help, or support and the grace with which he was able to accept all that his family and many friends gave. There was an endless supply of home-cooked meals in his room. He asked friends to stay with him when his wife needed to be away from his bedside. He was even able to respond to the sometimes convoluted messages of encouragement I would try to bring with me on my daily visits. He expertly organized the energies and efforts of his family, his friends, and his physicians on his behalf. This unique talent led him to plan, at a critical point in his course, to bring together several of the leading experts in bone marrow transplantation to offer a "consensus opinion" regarding his future medical management. He pointed out that decisions of far less magnitude were often handled in such a manner in the world of business or education. He never did convene this meeting of experts, but arrived at a very well-informed decision after much questioning and discussion.

Physicians can learn important lessons about coping with illness from patients like Saul. His strategy was to establish his own identity, to respond to the individual qualities of each person who cared for him, and to ask for and accept help. When I knew him better, I came to realize that these were precisely the qualities that had characterized his life before he became ill. I felt a certain satisfaction in thinking that my advice that first day had somehow made it easier for him to deal with his illness until I realized that my advice that he keep his jogging suit was not a product of my intuition; it was exactly what he was preparing to do. I had only responded to his cue! If that initial meeting helped Saul in any way, as I see it now, it was not my *advice* but rather the *recognition* of where his strengths lay that led me to encourage him to depend on those strengths. There is little advice we can give that can help patients to confront the existential fears associated with serious illness. Yet the desire to help, to support, to give something is very great. Most people have strengths which, if they can be used or mobilized, will sustain them and allow them to cope with what seem to be impossibly difficult conditions. Some patients declare their needs very openly and directly. More often we must rely on listening closely to the patient and learning more about their lives to understand their needs and find their strengths.

Richard was a successful chemical engineer and lifelong sailing enthusiast. He had sailed halfway round the world and was accustomed to being in control of his life, but his confidence in his strength was severely shaken when he developed, in rapid succession, an aggressive prostate cancer and myeloma. He confronted his initial treatments with determination but desperately needed some rational explanation in order to comprehend why, after a life of physical activity and careful attention to diet, he should have developed two different types of cancer. He had been a close friend for many years when he was well, vigorous, and active. I knew that early in his career as an engineer he had worked on the Atomic Energy Project. I recalled how he had described carrying in his arms "this radioactive material that actually glowed." I suggested that his cancers might possibly be related to this earlier heavy radiation exposure rather than to any weakness on his part. This idea, an unproven speculation at best, seemed to strike a resonant chord. He seemed to summon up his own strength to "fight back." He remained a formidable figure throughout his illness. I will never forget his response when another patient died in his four-bedded hospital room. Having watched, over several hours, as an intern cared for an elderly man who "went sour" and died, he called the young man to him later that day and commended the care and sensitivity he had displayed. Patients die of their illnesses, and Richard died of his. But before he died, he lived bravely and courageously, sharing every possible moment of hope with his equally strong and courageous wife. I would like to believe that our discussion of radiation and cancer risk helped him to face his terrible, and ultimately fatal, illnesses. I have no doubt that the discussion helped create a bond of understanding that made it easier for me to care for him.

Not all patients are so charismatic, so able to be strong or to control their lives. Some worry about all manner of symptoms, dwell on their seemingly trivial illnesses and voice the concern that they will not be able

34   to cope with the next illness. I did not know what to expect when I had to tell Ellen that she had a large malignant kidney tumor. She had come to me several years earlier for treatment of what was thought to be a very unusual metabolic disorder but proved to be self-induced electrolyte loss. I never fully confronted her with my diagnosis but, during the course of the next few years, she apparently abandoned her abuse of laxatives. She remained, in my mind, a fragile, unfulfilled, and unhappy woman. I was very cautious in presenting the difficult news that I had to deliver. I was quite unprepared for the matter-of-fact manner in which she heard her diagnosis and went through surgery. She sought out the most promising new approaches to immunotherapy in a forthright, almost aggressive way. She traveled across the country to seek an expert opinion. She was at once angry and challenging as she dealt with an illness that I had feared might paralyze her. She was rebellious and not easily intimidated. She undertook a difficult course of treatment and, in her own words, "bitched" when her tumor recurred, but she did not flinch, and she ploughed ahead with her treatment. In caring for her I came to realize that she had spent her entire life battling, in her unsuccessful career, within her family, and with illnesses, real and imagined. This illness, in a way, gave her the opportunity to enter and do battle openly and to demonstrate her courage and resolve.

An old medical adage says, Ask the patient, they will tell you what is wrong. I have learned that if you get close and listen carefully, they will also tell you where their strengths, however remote or unexpected, can be found.

Reassurance and the Warning on the Label

Doctors seem to have adopted a note of caution, like the warning on labels, in reassuring patients or families. Each measure of reassurance is accompanied by a carefully worded warning. Caveat emptor! We cannot really be certain, there is much we do not know . . ." This troubles me. What is there about reassurance that makes us feel the need to attach a warning label? And what are the consequences of this labeling?

Reassurance has always been an integral part of the physician's role in caring. At times the physician may have a clear understanding of the problem, and this knowledge may be sufficient to dispel uncertainty and to reassure without reservation. More often there is some uncertainty in the physician's mind so that the outcome is in doubt. The need of many patients and their families for reassurance is often very great and at times insatiable. It could be said that the "health hazard" of reassurance, given without qualification, is that it creates a false sense of security, false hopes. The pain of disappointment and dashed hopes is very great, and the anger that follows being misled or deceived can be bitter. In these times of increasing malpractice litigation, it is hard to be critical of physicians who, 35

36   in order to protect their patients and themselves, cautiously avoid unrealistic reassurance, painting an overly optimistic picture, or creating false hopes.[1] But these considerations only touch the surface of the issue of reassurance in the relationship between physicians and patients. Physicians feel the need to reassure as much as patients need to be reassured. It is part of the reward and pleasure that comes in caring for patients. On some level this represents a very old and fundamental interaction between physicians and patients, the physician's intuitive response to the anxiety, pain, uncertainty, and sense of loss expressed by patients.

If providing reassurance is such a natural urge among physicians, why do we find it hard to be reassuring to our patients and why are our reassurances so often carefully followed by disclaimers or warnings? In reaching for a response to this question, I think it is very important to draw a distinction between physicians' responses to the need for reassurance and the need for guidance or advice. I am fully aware of the considerable overlap. Real uncertainty, dealing with the unknown, limits our ability both to reassure and to give guidance or advice. Guidance in a setting of fear and anxiety may be reassuring and, conversely, reassurance often helps a patient to make difficult choices. Reassurance and advice overlap but differ in subtle though important ways and call upon very different strengths in the physician.

Consider what is involved in giving advice or guidance. For the physician this includes the very difficult tasks of choosing among therapeutic options and discussing prognosis and issues of quality of life. Physicians are acutely aware that many decisions are made in the face of great uncertainty. Some questions simply don't have a right answer. Increasingly we, both physicians and patients, seek data, published reports of studies, large or small, controlled or anecdotal, conclusive or only suggestive, for guidance. These represent systematic efforts to deal with uncertainty. Sometimes these studies provide clear evidence of the efficacy of a given treatment or the advantage of one treatment as compared with others and provide an assessment of the risks and side effects. A careful presentation of such information can do much to reduce the uncertainty and anxiety that patients experience when making difficult decisions.

That a proposed therapy has produced favorable results or has resulted in a   37
good prognosis can be very reassuring. More often, however, the conclusions to be drawn from published studies are not so clear-cut. How useful are the conflicting studies of treatment options in breast cancer published within the past few years to the physician who must recommend a specific treatment or to the woman faced with the choice of radical surgery, lumpectomy, chemotherapy, or radiation treatment? How are we to interpret the findings of the various large cooperative studies on the efficacy of coronary artery bypass surgery? Do they give clear guidance to the patient who is agonizing over the decision about whether to undergo this operation? Physicians trying to advise their patients, faced with difficult choices, do not find this an easy or straightforward task even when they are quite familiar with the results of such studies. Physicians sometimes say, "I tell them all the facts, and let them decide." Or "I allow the patient the autonomy to make a decision." We act as if the raw data will provide the answer and relieve us of responsibility. If you have ever listened to patients describe their discomfort with such advice or guidance, you will recognize that it simply doesn't work, by which I mean that it provides neither guidance nor support for a patient agonizing over a difficult choice. Second or third opinions occasionally help to resolve a problem; these opinions seem to be most helpful when they have been given by a physician in whom the patient feels greater trust or confidence. There is probably a considerable degree of wisdom in heeding these visceral responses in making difficult choices.

To fill the role of a knowledgeable advisor to the patient, the physician must be ready to critically evaluate the studies, to determine the degree to which the findings apply to the specific patient, and to interpret the findings and their significance for the patient. For decisions such as amniocentesis for prenatal diagnosis, organ donation for a family member, or HIV testing, the most important determinants in arriving at sound advice may be learned by listening to the patient's narrative and understanding the patient's values. In the end, it may be necessary to present a recommendation or advice that includes a caveat or warning reflecting the uncertainty behind the conclusion. "This appears to be the best

38 treatment at this time, but we do not yet know the long-term effects." This is still a far cry from today's common practice of appending a litany of every conceivable unpleasant outcome that might occur.

We often confuse the call for reassurance with a request for advice or guidance. We respond as though we had been asked for advice or guidance and speak of statistics and probabilities. We carefully qualify our reassurance—we affix a warning label. This is a mistake. A warning label is quite appropriate when attached to advice, but it seems out of place when the intent of the message is reassurance. This confusion comes about, in part, because of ambiguities in our use of language. When I ask a patient in my waiting room, "How are you?" it is a form of greeting. When I ask the same question, now as an inquiry, just a few minutes later in my consultation room, the response is usually quite different. Is it a call for reassurance or advice when the patient asks, "What will happen now?" or "How will I get through this?"

Providing reassurance is often much more difficult than giving advice, guidance, and counsel. When the diagnosis is clear-cut, the condition benign, self-limited, or curable, and the prognosis excellent, then it is easy to reassure. Often, however, it is apparent to both the physician and the patient that the outcome cannot be predicted or that the prognosis is, in fact, very poor. This situation is painful for both the physician and the patient. A colleague recently confided that he felt acutely uncomfortable with a patient, who had cancer, and her husband because "They hung so much on every word, looking for reassurance." He explained, "I just try to keep it light with them . . . at least it seems to help me." How can the physician give reassurance or encouragement when the patient has AIDS, advanced cancer, or Alzheimer's disease? When we know that the need for reassurance is great, how are we to respond?

Having struggled with some of these issues for almost thirty years, I have learned that the need for reassurance under these circumstances calls for the physician to use his or her relationship with the patient, rather than a measured guarded assessment, to provide support. The more uncertain the future and the bleaker the prognosis, the greater is the need for the support that can come from knowing that an educated caring physician is fully committed to seeing them through their illness, in a word, "being there." This is reassurance. The patient's call for reassurance is not a call for magic, miracles, or omniscience. It is a cry for a human connection. Reassurances that pain will be controlled, that dignity will be preserved, that the patient's wishes will be respected, and that the patient will not be left to face death alone require a significant commitment from a caring physician and do not require a warning label.

Defending the Common Cold

Medical science is on the verge of developing a vaccine and probably a cure for the common cold. The technical capability exists, there is a strong economic motivation, and at least one vaccine has already been tested. This is hailed as progress and an achievement of modern medicine. I disagree. My objections, which I will express even as I sit here sneezing and sniffling, might be framed in the context of the new Darwinian or evolutionary biology, which has gained some interest and favor lately. The Rhinovirus class, to which the common cold virus belongs, has its origins in prehistory. The doctrine of Darwinian biology suggests that there is some reason for the survival of this virus, in the face of the pressures of mutation and "survival of the fittest." I will not speculate about what made the cold virus so adept at survival during the millennia of its existence.

Speaking as the virus' host, I would like to go on record as stating, unequivocally, that there are some very good things about the common cold which make me ambivalent to the news of a cold vaccine. For the

sufferer, one of the best things about the common cold is that it is so easily diagnosed and is not easily confused with any other more serious or dangerous illnesses. Everyone knows that the prognosis for recovery from the common cold is excellent. When you get a common cold, you can be pretty sure that you will be well again soon without any lingering disability. Even singers, actors, and bassoonists, who are greatly inconvenienced by the common cold, know that they will recover fully. One of the best features of the common cold is that the sufferer will be easily diagnosed by those around him or her. The bleary eyes, the sneezing, and the red, runny nose are easily identified and usually evoke genuine sympathy. What other condition calls forth blessings ("Bless you," "Gesundheit") from total strangers? Contrast this with the many other illnesses that cause much greater suffering and have much more uncertain outcomes, but for which we get no sympathy at all because we do not *look* ill.

From the physician's side, the common cold is an ideal illness. First, the ease with which we can diagnose the malady, even from a description of the symptoms given over the telephone, confirms our diagnostic abilities. Consider how we make the diagnosis. We rely almost exclusively on the patient's history and our physical examination to diagnose the common cold. Though tissue culture and virologic studies could be employed to the isolate, identify, and classify the Rhinovirus, we are comfortable making the diagnosis on clinical grounds alone. In the present climate of defensive medicine, one rarely hears of the need to perform additional testing "just to be sure." Even further, because we have always known (that is, even before our medical training) that the prognosis is good, we are able to suppress the fear that a common cold can "get into the chest" and become pneumonia. We offer hot tea, chicken soup, and reassurance without a warning label. As I recall the many phone conversations I have had with patients with colds, I think the element of shared responsibility and care is fairly unique. The patient generally knows what can be done and calls only for reassurance and confirmation. The physician is able, with honesty, to acknowledge that the outcome is not in her or his hands and at the same time to be reassuring.

I can hear my reader's bemused question: What can consideration of such a simple affliction teach us about dealing with more serious illnesses?

42   The oft-heard criticism, "If medicine cannot find the cure for the common cold, how will it find a cure for cancer?" assumes that the common cold should be easily comprehended because it is a mild, benign illness. The truth of the matter is that the interaction between the cold virus and its human host has much to teach about the pathogenesis of cancer. Similarly, although the common cold is a minor, self-limited affair, almost more of an inconvenience than an illness, there are aspects of physicians' responses to the common cold that might serve as a paradigm for responses to other, more serious or even life-threatening illnesses.

Consider a migraine headache. Severe headaches may be disabling and, for the sufferer, often evoke deep fears of brain tumor, cerebral hemorrhage, or meningitis. As with the common cold, close attention to the patient's description of the typical symptoms of unilateral, throbbing pain often associated with nausea and with visual symptoms such as light flashes, zig-zag distortions, and even blind spots allows the physician to be relatively confident of the diagnosis of migraine headache. Eliciting a history of prior, similar headaches makes this diagnosis fairly certain without a need to resort to a host of very frightening and costly diagnostic tests to rule out more serious pathology. As with the common cold, patients who have experienced recurrent migraine headaches phone their physician, at times, simply to confirm their own diagnosis and to be reassured. Although the immediate disability may be great, the prognosis is excellent. Since the treatments for migraine are more effective than tea or chicken soup, the physician can offer both effective treatment and reassurance.

Finally, I would like to examine the thesis that the common cold can teach us something about an illness for which pathophysiology and diagnostic accuracy are well developed, such as coronary artery disease and anginal syndrome. Complaints of chest pain or substernal pressure are common in patients with established coronary artery disease. The patient may have had a previously documented myocardial infarction and may even have had coronary angiography which documented, in frightening detail, the extent of coronary artery lesions. The physician's assessment of any given episode of chest discomfort or pain, often described by a worried patient over the phone, calls for close listening to the patient's description of the symptoms. Even the most cautious physician does not recommend that each time a patient calls with such a complaint they report immediately to an emergency room or come to the office for an electrocardiogram. Some calls to the physician to describe chest discomfort seem to be like the calls from patients with the common cold. The patient does not think he is having a heart attack but calls for confirmation and some measure of reassurance. As with the common cold or migraine headache there are clues in the patient's narrative that are very useful in making this assessment. Patients who have experienced many episodes of chest pressure or pain for which they did not call their physician or go to the hospital emergency room, somehow recognize when their symptoms are more serious and warrant immediate attention. Unlike the common cold or migraine headache, there are tests that would establish a positive diagnosis of myocardial infarction, but the evidence is quite good that the physicians' diagnostic accuracy, using the history alone, is comparable to the precision of much more elaborate diagnostic methods.[1] Despite the formidable understanding of the etiology and pathophysiology of angina and myocardial infarction that we have derived from cellular and molecular biology, the physician's role in caring for the patient with angina or a heart attack has much in common with his or her role in caring for the patient with migraine headaches or many other illnesses, including the common cold.

But back to the Rhinovirus. Perhaps it will be discovered that infection with the common cold virus confers protection against other more virulent infectious agents. The evolutionary biologists will hail this as an important discovery, and those who are busy developing a vaccine against the common cold will have to reconsider the possible negative consequences of their efforts. If a successful vaccine is produced, I will consider it a mixed blessing, because it seems that the common cold can teach us much about being a physician and about physician-patient relations.

Asymmetry

The uncertainty, fear of loss, and helplessness experienced by patients are mirrored in the responses of their physicians. This is an empathic response triggered by the patient's suffering or anguish. But it is also a direct response to uncertainty, to the awesome responsibilities involved in the physician's role, and to the threatening awareness of the inevitability of illness and loss that we all feel. Although these emotional responses are shared by physicians and patients, the sharing is asymmetric. The plain fact is that the patient and the patient's family always suffer more than the physician. Whether giving a simple injection or a piece of bad news, the physician can never honestly assert, "This hurts me as much as it hurts you." Serious illness is often the central issue in the thoughts, feelings, and day-to-day lives of patients. Sheila Rothman, describing the narratives of patients with tuberculosis wrote, "Several themes cut across all these encounters with illness and are of especial importance to understanding the patient experience. First was the challenge that uncertainty posed for the sick, their families and their doctors . . . there was no way of knowing whether a remission might last for months, years or decades. Lives were lived in the shadow of the disease, as decisions had to be made about careers, about marriage, and about childbearing."[1]

What does it mean to conclude that the relationship between patient and physician is asymmetric? Clearly, just because the injection, the bad news, or the illness cause more pain for the patient than for the physician does not imply that the physician is insensitive to the patient's experience. Symmetry is not a realistic expectation and is not, in any way, a criterion for a good physician-patient relationship. The asymmetry in physician and patient responses is not simply quantitative. It does not rest on the fulcrum of who suffers or feels more. The responses of the patient and of the physician are both conditioned by a lifetime of earlier experiences. For the physician, the emotional response to one patient's illness merges with responses to the pain and losses shared with many patients, current and past. The cumulative effect on the physician may be very great. I doubt that many medical students think about this. I know that it was not something I thought about as a young physician. I suppose my awareness of this aspect of the asymmetric relationship between patients and physicians, the cumulative weight of much suffering and many losses, began early in my career when an older physician asked if I would be willing, over a period of time, to take over the care of some of his patients. He was a very highly regarded internist, renowned as a master clinician and credited with several original observations in clinical medicine. Although still active and vigorous, he explained that he was beginning to find it difficult to deal with serious, often fatal illnesses of patients who had been under his care since he, and they, had escaped from Europe at the start of World War II. I was honored by his request and I readily agreed, but we did not discuss his feelings any further. He referred only one or two patients from his very active practice before he died.

Thinking back to that experience almost thirty years ago has led me to ponder how physicians deal with the cumulative weight of the many asymmetric relationships in their lives. Medical care has become more intense and places a great responsibility on physicians who, though they may be highly specialized, function as the primary physicians for their patients. I have often experienced this in my role as a nephrologist and

46   internist, but I suspect that many of my colleagues who specialize in fields such as oncology, AIDS, degenerative neurologic diseases, or pediatric neurosurgery, to name only a few, must experience this uncertainty, loss, and grief every day. How do they deal with the cumulative weight of these heavy emotional demands? In my experience, these are not subjects that my colleagues in medicine readily discuss.

Realizing this, I decided to interview several of my colleagues to see whether I could learn more about how some other physicians cope. I chose physicians who, to my mind, bore very great patient responsibilities and dealt with complex, life-threatening illnesses. I selected individuals who seemed to be very good at what they did, thinking that there might be lessons to be learned by listening to their narratives.

There were some common threads, but for the most part, as with patients' narratives, theirs were unique, compelling, and instructive but did not lend themselves to generalizations. Bits of conversations, anecdotes, and observations linger in my mind.

Dr. Jeff Greene was completing his fellowship in infectious disease when the strange, fatal illness, today known as AIDS, made its appearance in New York City. Jeff became one of the first clinical AIDS researchers and is today a leading physician in the field. He describes himself as "an AIDS doc." It was clear to me that, apart from his extensive knowledge of AIDS, Jeff knew his patients well. He knew a great deal about their lives, their needs, their families, and their partners. He admired the courage which led many of his HIV-infected patients to continue to pursue creative lives and meaningful personal relationships. He made house calls to see terminally ill patients too weak to leave home. "It is amazing to look at a 78-pound skeleton of a man and see that he has around him barbells, photographs, and paintings that are reminders of his life." Jeff long ago became reconciled to the fact that virtually all his patients will die of their disease. "It gives me a good feeling when I think of the thousands of man-hours I have helped patients to enjoy." He does not often attend memorials, funerals, or pay condolence calls.

Dr. Fred Epstein, a world-class pediatric neurosurgeon, deals almost exclusively with tumors of the brain stem and spinal cord. As I sat in his

waiting room, I could not help noticing that the atmosphere was friendly
and not at all somber, though the families and children I observed were
serious and concerned. Fred's office is filled with photographs of his
family, memorabilia, and poignant notes from grateful patients and families. The "magnetic center" of his office is not the desk or X-ray view
box, but a large couch and several comfortable chairs. Each week he talks
with at least six families who must learn that their child has an incurable,
probably fatal, condition. "Sometimes along with the sick child and the
parents there may be siblings and one or two sets of grandparents. You've
got to get a whole family through something. You never lose the sense of
the cataclysm that they are experiencing. It is emotionally draining because of the magnitude."

He showed me some of the letters he had received in the past few
weeks. "This is one of the things that buoy me up. I often get letters, even
years later, from families whose children have died. . . . We lose 30
percent of our patients, 30 percent. They tell me that we've helped them
survive something that was not a survivable situation. You have to do
something that helps them find the resources to get through it. I go to the
home sometimes. I get asked the damndest questions like, What is death?
and Am I going to die?" When I asked what he says to a dying child or to
the family, his answer was simple and direct, "Nothing, they know. I am
just there, and I let them know I am there."

Though he has an international reputation as an outstanding pediatric
neurosurgeon, Fred was unequivocal in assessing his role. "Fifty years ago
there were a few unique geniuses in the field. Today the aura and the
mystique are gone. I can train anyone to be a good surgeon. When they
are finished, in a year or two, they will be as good as I am. I don't come
out of the O.R. saying, 'God, I did that well!' I am trained to do these
operations. After surgery I often explain, 'We just don't know. We are just
people together. We want the best thing for our kids.' The difference is
how you help families, how you get them through it."

I knew Dr. Edwin Kolodny when he was a medical student and I was
resident or a young attending in medicine. He returned to New York
University Medical Center, as chairman of the department of neurology,

48 having made major contributions to the detection and understanding of Tay-Sachs disease and several heritable neurodegenerative diseases. A career dedicated to the care of children or young adults with progressive neurologic disorders epitomized for me the meaning of a cumulative burden of pain and loss. What I heard from Ed was a description of a life that was full, rich, and rewarding. He seemed to be nourished by his deep religious convictions, by his active involvement in elucidating the nature of the diseases he treats, and by his own strong sense of family. "Every patient teaches me something. We are in this together, both getting something out of the encounter. Patients and families often come to me, angry and hurt, having been told 'This is the diagnosis, there is nothing we can do.' After examining the child and all the information they have brought, I usually say, 'Every child is different. We will have to see together what will happen.' I am happy if I can make someone more comfortable with their disease. Helping families is a great source of satisfaction. I also have the research lab to fall back on. I am excited by going to the lab and coming back with an answer."

He described relationships with some patients that had extended over many years. In some instances, in what I regard as the most profound validation of the relationship, families or patients requested that he perform an autopsy examination to advance science's understanding of their disease.

Dr. Martin Kahn is an outstanding clinical cardiologist. I have had many chances to witness the extraordinarily thorough and sensitive care he gives to patients. In an era in which cardiologists have subspecialized, and in a field that is increasingly guided by technology, Marty has remained a dedicated, well-informed clinician-cardiologist. I had a sense that his practice, aside from his many teaching commitments at New York University, was very demanding. I was not fully prepared for his description of the frequency of emergencies, the volume of data, and the number of phone calls he must respond to each day. He explained, "It is painful to realize that many of my patients were my present age when I first started treating them fifteen or twenty years ago. Now their medical problems are becoming increasingly complex and debilitating. These

patients are now quite fragile and their clinical course unpredictable.
They require frequent visits for lab tests and medication changes. Any additional medical problem introduces new complexities and dangers. Even a small change in potassium level or blood clotting could become life-threatening if not attended to promptly. The immediacy of the current practice of cardiology can be overwhelming."

Although Marty clearly values and enjoys his role as the primary physician for a number of his cardiac patients, he acknowledged that being deeply involved with many patients, on a personal and technical level, contributed to the need for some coping strategy. He concluded, "I think the most important component of my coping is being part of a larger organization that shares my goals. The medical center provides an environment where I can continue my education and help educate students and house staff. It allows easy access to colleagues with great expertise and commitment." To my ear Marty was describing being renewed by a "midnight meal" consisting of an ongoing chain of meetings with colleagues and students.

Dr. Machelle Allen, an obstetrician-gynecologist, is responsible for the Special Prenatal Program, a clinic for pregnant substance-abusing and HIV-positive women at Bellevue Hospital. She described herself as "a product of the sixties." With an interest in primary care, she was drawn to women's health; several years after she completed her training, she began to focus her attention on chemically-dependent and seropositive women. Although I envisioned this to be an impossibly demanding and painful way of life for a physician, medical students who had spent elective periods with Dr. Allen praised her commitment and sensitivity.[2] It was evident that the great burden of responsibility in caring for women with the full gamut of social problems that accompany drug-dependence and HIV infection could not rest on one individual. The Special Prenatal Program, which includes a nurse, social worker, domestic violence counselor and advocate, HIV counselor, and obstetrician, provides an important model for the care of complex and demanding medical and social problems. Machelle explained that she, and the patients, coped by focusing on short-term goals. HIV-infected women who are pregnant are

50   generally not yet ill with full-blown AIDS. Their major concerns, as with all pregnant women, are related to the health of their babies. "A woman was human before she was HIV-infected or chemically dependent." For Machelle, "My gratification derives from having had an impact on someone's life—from seeing a patient come to term, not preterm, drug-free—and from seeing the woman pleased with herself." She explained that it was important that she keep her goals short-term, acknowledging the high rate of recidivism among drug-dependent patients.

There were some common themes among these narratives. As I expected, all agreed that these were not issues that were often discussed with other physicians, family, or friends. Perhaps the strongest recurrent theme was the feeling that there was "not enough time." Machelle Allen smiled as she said, "It has been so long since I finished my work in a day." Ed Kolodny noted that setting "priorities for time can be unbearable." Fred Epstein described how he regularly took a suitcase of X-rays home and often returned phone calls between 10 P.M. and midnight; "It's manageable, but every minute is taken." He related an incident that occurred seven or eight years earlier: "The mother of a patient I had known for a long time called me aside and said, 'Let me tell you something. You are not spending time with patients as you used to. You are moving too fast.' I listened to her. She shocked me, and I was grateful for that." This led to Fred's recruiting an additional pediatric neurosurgeon into the program. Yet this was the exception. The other physicians with whom I spoke did not foresee a way to reduce the time pressures they experienced, but generally expressed the belief that "things were under [their] control." As I listened to my colleagues speak of dealing with these time pressures, I sensed that I was hearing a deeper, unarticulated theme, that of experiencing the pain and suffering of their patients. I know that full commitment to the care of patients who are ill places impossible demands on the time and energies of physicians. It is no surprise that it is easier for us to articulate and discuss the time pressures than to confront the more existential pain and fears we experience. The real value in this substitution is apparent when my colleagues explain that they feel satisfied when they "have things under control." Demands on time can be dealt with by prioritizing and careful managing one's schedule. Dealing with the demands made on one's emotional strengths and energies is not so easy. I question the formulation "control of the demands on my time leads to satisfaction." I wonder whether the feeling of "control" truly leads to satisfaction. I suspect that it might be the other way around. I had the sense that each of these physicians derived great satisfaction from the human connections with patients and families that each of them had described in strong personal terms. My own reaction, and my sense of what I had learned from these colleagues (if these can be separated), is that their rewarding clinical experiences made the intense time pressures acceptable and left each physician with the sense that "things were under control" or "manageable."

I did not find a clear answer to the question, How do these physicians deal with the cumulative uncertainty, loss, and grief? In the end, it seems to me that physicians cope with this burden of grief and uncertainty in the same ways that patients deal with their individual suffering. As is the case with some patients, some physicians deal poorly. They experience burnout; they express dysphoria, anger, cynicism; they resort to "psychic numbing," to alcohol and drugs. More often, however, they draw on their own strengths and coping mechanisms. My brief survey of a highly selected group of my colleagues served to confirm my long-held belief that the sense of renewal and gratification that physicians derive from the experience of responsive and compassionate relationships with patients probably provides the greatest counterweight to the cumulative burden of uncertainty, grief, and loss.

On Drawing Blood

"I had to take blood from my patient. She asked whether I had done this before. I said I had, but I didn't tell her that it was only once, or that it was on a man with *great* veins. I knew it was important for me to do it." This was a medical student, early in his first clinical rotation, opening a discussion among a small group of classmates. I listened as the student described his hesitance, his clumsiness, his initial unsuccessful efforts at venipuncture, and finally his triumphal "stab." I noted how his tentative opening remark drew out similar descriptions from the others in the group and, as the discussion went on, I realized that while I was hearing the anecdotes, I was responding to a deeper undertone. I was reminded of the experience of recognizing a familiar folk theme in a symphony or a string quartet. I found myself listening to the "ground bass" as the students, one by one, described their experiences and responses to the seemingly inconsequential act of drawing blood from a patient. Inconsequential? I am sure both the students and most of their teachers would see this skill as but a small part of the mass of more complex skills and information that students acquire during the clinical years in medical school. But like

the folk theme that keeps repeating in some place between your ear and
your mind, my thoughts returned again and again to many hour-long
discussions of some aspect of drawing blood from patients. I began to see
that this "inconsequential" task had a deeper significance, that drawing
blood represented, in a microcosm, many very important aspects of the
student's entry into the world of doctoring.

Although medical school curricula provide students with the opportunity to meet patients in the first and second years in order to learn the
skills of patient interviewing or physical diagnosis, these meetings do not
approximate the doctor-patient relationship. The clearly stated goals of
the "clinical years" are to develop the manual skills and to acquire the
knowledge critical for the care of patients, yet the setting of the clinical
clerkship places the medical student squarely in a physician-patient relationship. The medical student may introduce himself or herself to the
patient as a student, a clinical clerk, or a clinical associate, but the student
and the patient invariably experience the relationship as that of physician
and patient. How can the student assume this new role? Others, the
interns, the resident, the supervising physician, or the private attending
physician, know more medicine and are more directly responsible for the
care of the patient. For the student, the unique role in doctoring comes
with the requirement to draw blood. This responsibility, generally considered a "noneducational task" or "scut work," is in fact the way in
which learning the doctor-patient relationship often begins. Although
the builders of Notre Dame might have been thinking of the rose win-
dows, the actual work began with mixing cement and chipping stones.
We can structure the education of medical students in the preclinical
years as a systematic layering of interrelated facts and principles, but
the educational experience in the clinical years is unpredictable because it
is patient-centered. For many students this first contact with serious
illness and suffering is very frightening. For the novice clinical clerk, it
requires some accessible point of entry. Drawing blood is the entry point
for many students. Full-time phlebotomists routinely draw blood for tests
every morning in most hospitals, but when a medical student performs
the same "routine" venipuncture it comes to embody many important

54 components of the physician-patient relationship. Centrally it is an act that brings the student and patient into physical contact. Touching is no simple matter for many students, and this physical contact differs from a handshake or a brief pat on the shoulder. It is more prolonged and deliberate and is often followed by a judgment. Will the patient say, "You have a light touch," or "I barely felt it," or "I felt you digging around"? In most instances the physical contact involved in drawing blood is, for the student and the patient, a relatively safe contact in that it does not require the patient to disrobe or to be exposed.[1] Not every patient submits willingly to having blood taken by a medical student. For the medical student, the task of drawing blood may require a preliminary building of trust ("I'm quite good at this and you have excellent veins") or even a lengthy explanation of the reasons for performing the blood test and the possible interpretations or consequences of the results of the test. Since medical students are involved in the care of the patients, they feel compelled to respond to these questions. These conversations represent one way that the student progresses beyond the entry point in the physician-patient relationship. The important issues of building trust and maintaining honesty are evident even in these brief encounters.

When a patient has been subjected to frequent venipunctures, additional blood drawing may require a degree of "negotiation" between the medical student and the patient. Whether the patient is a recidivist drug abuser with endocarditis or a frightened and frail elderly patient, the student drawing blood may be called upon to define the importance of each "stick" and, in doing so, to clarify the expectations and obligations of the physician-patient relationship. I have frequently heard students describe their discomfort when patients ask questions that they cannot answer. Patients may ask for information that is not available, they may question the judgment of the physician directing their care, and they may sometimes express their painful, existential fears. The entry point can be like the lid of Pandora's Box!

Discussions of experiences related to venipuncture frequently occupy whole sessions of our Humanistic Medicine group meetings with students. These are "critical incidents"[2] that students use, consciously or not, as an entry point from which they can explore their own feelings 55 about many other aspects of contact with patients. These experiences are critical in the development of young physicians. If I have identified a true "folk theme" in their narratives, blood drawing should be considered a very important, and undervalued, step in the early development of our medical students. Blood-drawing teams, nurse-practitioners, and physician's assistants are often thought of as a means of freeing up physicians to care for patients, but we should not lose sight of what may be lost in "freeing" students from the "noneducational task" of drawing blood. The process of becoming a physician is not one particularly suited to streamlining, efficiency, or standardization. Some of the most formative and important aspects of the process are unplanned and often, like drawing blood, unrecognized by medical educators.

The Vital Signs

Probably nothing generates more feelings of awkwardness, uncertainty, and anxiety in medical students than the introduction to physical examination. This is readily understandable. Most initial person-to-person contacts are fraught with tension for both parties, especially the earliest encounters between medical students and patients, which carry deep undertones related to vulnerability, intimacy, and privacy.

It is not simply the awkwardness that students experience in performing the manual tasks of palpation, percussion or auscultation. Medical students traditionally practice these techniques on their colleagues, and beyond a measure of self-consciousness, these techniques do not evoke the much more unsettling feelings that attend the examination of a patient. It is for this reason that the physical examination, which is so much more than inspection, palpation, percussion, and auscultation, must ultimately be learned by examining patients rather than colleagues or surrogates.

Physical examination, while providing much information for the examiner, also represents an important interaction between the examiner

and the patient. Physical examination is one of the languages of medicine.
While the physical examination tells the physician much about the patient, it also communicates a great deal to the patient. During physical
examination, as during the patient interview, the interaction involves all
the components of the physician-patient relationship. The part of the
examination that poses the greatest problem for many of us is clearly
inspection or observation. It is the most exposed part of the encounter
with the patient. There is a natural tendency to hide the discomfort at the
start of an examination by proceeding quickly to the parts of the examination that feel less threatening, for example, measuring blood pressure
or counting the pulse rate. Inspection and observation are powerful tools,
but their proper application requires definite preparation. In part, this
preparation takes the form of developing awareness of important cues or
signals. Odors, bedside photographs, the patient's gestures and body language, and the emotional tone of the initial greeting reveal much about
the patient and help to bridge the uncomfortable gap between the student or physician and the patient. Physical examination requires touching. All societies and cultures define the limits of acceptable physical contact very precisely. Handshakes, embraces, and touching, in the absence
of intimacy, are generally highly stylized and precisely defined. Physical
examination crosses many of the usual societal boundaries, though the
forms of contact in the course of physical examination are also fairly
precisely delimited. Physical examination requires the patient's trust. It
might be assumed that the patient implicitly expresses trust by agreeing to
the examination, but in fact, the trust develops during the course of the
examination as the patient responds to the gestures, questions, and touch
of the examiner. There is no simple formula for creating this trust. The
first step requires the examiner to be attentive to the person as an individual, not simply to the medical problem at issue. Patients look for this
recognition. Trust grows as the patient recognizes that the examiner has
been attentive and has responded with sensitivity to important signals in
the form of a spoken or unspoken word or phrase, a gesture, or a wince as
the examiner's hand approaches a tender area.

Issues of patient anxiety and the need for reassurance surface during

58   the physical examination. Every student and physician develops his or her own style. What seems most important is that from the earliest contact with patients, the student recognize that learning physical examination involves not only the acquisition of manual or technical skills directed at developing a data base or eliciting abnormal findings but also the development of an awareness of the multilayered interaction that takes place during even the most noninvasive aspects of physical examination.

It seems to me that medical students might do well to begin by carefully observing "the vital signs"—skin temperature, heart rate, and rate of breathing. For hospitalized patients, a record is regularly made of TPR (temperature, pulse, and respiration). This is not a technical exercise. Monitoring devices in most modern hospitals provide a very accurate, continuous digital display of the heart rate and rhythm, the respiratory rate (and even the depth and regularity of breathing), and the temperature at multiple skin sites. The physical skills required to examine the arterial pulse, respiration, and skin temperature are simple and easily learned. More important is the fact that preparation for this portion of the examination should lead the student to consider the question, What information can be gained from examining the vital signs? The vital signs, more than any other part of the physical examination or any laboratory test reflect much about the patient's level of anxiety; cardiac, circulatory, and lung function; and the activity of the autonomic nervous system. When the ability of the heart to pump blood is impaired, sympathetic nervous activity maintains cardiac output by increasing the heart rate and supports arterial blood pressure by constricting vessels. The resultant weak, rapid pulse with cool hands and feet may be important signs of impaired cardiac function, either cardiac or circulatory failure. Changes in pulse rate and the force of the pulse with minor exertion serve as a bedside stress test. Much can be learned simply by watching the patient breathe, but normal respiration is almost unapparent to both the patient and the examiner and requires close observation. The assessment of skin temperature, by touch, is dependent on the perception of a temperature gradient between the skin of the examiner and that of the patient. Though we have a variety of electronic devices and heat-sensitive color indicators to measure skin temperature, few are as sensitive as the mother's lips against the child's 59 forehead. It should be clear to the reader at this point that I view the assessment of the vital signs not as a narrow introduction to physical diagnosis but rather as a very rich source of information about the patient's health. This examination encompasses much of what is performed by shamans, healers, and Eastern physicians.[1] Although the technology of medicine has progressed so that many important body functions can be measured and monitored electronically, each medical student begins at the same point as the generations of physicians which preceded him or her. Assessment of the vital signs, the most noninvasive aspect of physical examination, has always been an important first step.

The Dummy and the Standardized Patient

The medical resident, visibly upset, arrived late to our meeting. Usually an active member of the group, today he remained silent, and his silence created a heaviness in the room. I felt a sense of relief when he began to explain, "I would like to describe what happened on my way here." He went on to explain that this week he was the medical resident responsible for supervising emergency treatment when a patient anywhere in the hospital suffered a cardiac arrest and required resuscitation. This is termed, "running the code." On his way to our conference, his beeper went off, and he was summoned for a "code." The elevator seemed to take forever. He got off and ran down the hallway to the patient's room. He arrived to find a nursing supervisor holding a stop watch. Several other house physicians were standing beside the plastic model which was used to test resuscitation skills. "I recognized that this was a test, and I was informed that it had taken me too long to arrive. I was angry; it wasn't my fault that the elevators take forever in this place. My job was to organize the team for the resuscitation, to 'run the code.'

The model is programmed to generate different heart rhythms and blood

pressures, and my job is to respond by ordering the correct medications, 61
to administer external cardiac compression, and to apply electrical shock
(cardioversion) if indicated." I settled back, listening to his description of
this experience, thankful I had never been in such a situation. "It is a real
challenge, you get totally involved in saving this dummy, making certain
that everyone is doing their job. I knew it was only a dummy and that it
was only a test, but that didn't seem to matter. When it was over, the
supervisor who had been watching, timing, and checking things off on a
list, said we had done well, and I was very relieved. Then . . . ." He looked
around the room with a pained expression. "I realized that I had put more
effort into 'saving' the damn dummy than I had with any code on a live
person. What is happening to me, and what kind of doctor am I becoming?" I believe we all shared the pain he felt in seeing his self-image as a
caring physician challenged by this experience, but I don't think his
response to the test situation was in any way unusual. I had no question
that he was more concerned with people than with dummies or tests.
The incident, however, seems to connect in my mind with other circumstances in which teaching medicine seems to have been dissociated from
the care of the patient. A striking example is the monthly student clinico-
pathologic conference (CPC). This traditional teaching exercise presents
students with a description of selected details of a patient's history, physical findings, laboratory results, and course of illness. By tradition, the case
history presented is that of an actual patient. The students are expected to
study the details and arrive at a diagnosis, which they submit, in writing,
before the CPC conference. Several students are called upon to defend
the diagnoses they have submitted. The CPC invariably generates a great
deal of intellectual activity among students and house staff. Journal references are tracked down and read with care, statistics are quoted, and
heated discussions take place among students, house staff, and attending
physicians. All agree that the CPC is very instructive and seems to engage
the minds of the students and house staff more than most other conferences. However this is precisely the aspect which troubles me, just as
our resident was upset by the intensity of his response to "saving the
dummy." I know that some of the patients under the care of these same

62 physicians pose diagnostic problems as challenging and puzzling as the patients described in the CPC, but rarely do their cases stimulate the same intellectual activity. I frankly deplore the fact that so much more effort, thought, and emotion is directed at the CPC patient than at the living patient "in the next bed," but I have come to understand the phenomenon.

The CPC exercise is stripped of "extraneous details," such as the patient's fears and concerns, the demands of the family, the pressure to treat, and considerations of patients' complaints or finances. It is precisely, at least in part, because the CPC is stripped of "these extraneous details" that it can engage our full intellectual energies and provide an interesting and instructive exercise. It represents an opportunity to consider a very wide range of diagnostic possibilities, even some which are very rare or exotic, without risk to the patient. Even the most challenging CPC cannot approach the rich experience and rewards of patient care, but there is no question that diagnosing and treating the real patient are far more demanding and difficult.

In medical education, growing use is made of selected readings and videotape interviews in teaching medical students and house staff about patients' responses to illness, coping mechanisms, and other "humanistic" aspects of medicine. I have mixed feelings about this. There is no question that artists have always been uniquely able to heighten our awareness and responses to all aspects of the human condition. Powerful, evocative descriptions of patients suffering from all manner of ills can be found in writing, dance, music, and the graphic arts. Stories can teach all of us much that is relevant to the patients under our care. Equally, the stories and words of our patients and students carry important messages and lessons. For me, few literary pieces have been as moving or instructive as the lessons I have learned firsthand from my patients or students. But that is not the critical issue. Both literary descriptions and the words and stories of our patients can sensitize and teach us if we listen for their real content, rather than as the form in which the patient presents his "chief complaint and present illness."

Most of all I am concerned about the recent introduction of the "standardized clinical examination," which makes use of simulated pa-

tients, actors or actresses skilled in the presentation of a set of complaints   63
and even capable of simulating abnormal physical findings. The format of
the examination, requiring that the student approach the "standardized
patient" and inquire about initial complaints and symptoms and the "patient's" response to illness, is based on pretense. Though I recognize the
goals and the merit behind attempting to achieve some uniformity or
standardization in evaluating medical students, the pretense troubles me.
An evaluation of performance, which tacitly accepts that the physician-
patient interaction is actually a dialogue between an actor playing a patient and a physician (student) acting a part, presents our students with a
message that is worse than distorted. I wonder whether the thinking
behind the introduction of a "standardized patient" for *evaluation* will lead
to the introduction of "standardized patients" for *teaching* medicine or, in
my worst-case scenario, to the development of a "standardized medical
role model." In a way, the dummy that is used to teach cardiopulmonary
resuscitation can be viewed as a "standardized patient." Admittedly, this is
a highly effective tool for preparing physicians, nurses, and emergency
medical technicians to treat patients who have suffered cardiac or respiratory arrest. Considering the technology involved and the urgent nature
of the problem, the dummy is precisely what is required to teach, in a safe
and controlled fashion, how to deal with life-or-death cardiac arrest. It is
not intended to provide the student with insight into whom to resusci-
tate, when to stop, and how to deal with the emotional issues that students and house staff experience during and after participation in a
"code." That is our responsibility as teachers.

Technology is attractive. It can be "standardized," it is cost-effective,
reproducible, and portable. Actors and actresses may simulate symptoms
and signs and give very instructive feedback to students. Heart sound
simulators can reproduce heart murmurs, rubs, and gallops with great
fidelity, and are wonderful tools for teaching physical diagnosis. Computer programs allow the student to "dissect" a cadaver, layer by layer,
without experiencing the offensive odor of formaldehyde. And yet it is
clear to any of us who teach medical students or young physicians that
these tools can never replace the patient-centered forms of teaching that

64   have been the traditional mainstay of medical education. I strongly suspect this reflects the fact that what is taught (and learned) when a student
dissects the brachial plexus, listens to a patient's heart, or hears the medical history is not easily captured by a computer program, a high fidelity
sound generator, or a programmed dummy.

Holding the Blood Gas Report

The student, who was midway through his clerkship in medicine, had been a quiet listener during most of our weekly group meetings. On this afternoon, he broke a lengthy period of silence by stating simply, "Something upset me yesterday." He explained that during this, his first clinical clerkship, he had been present at several attempted bedside cardiac resuscitations. He explained that each time he stood by and watched the medical residents and interns perform the various maneuvers of cardiopulmonary resuscitation, he felt acutely uncomfortable because "things moved so fast" that he felt he could not be of any help. "Yesterday," he went on, "the team was called for a code on one of my patients. We rushed to the bedside and the house staff began to intubate him and start chest compression. In the middle of everything the intern handed a syringe of blood to me and told me to get an arterial blood gas." He rushed out of the room, brought the blood sample to a laboratory on the next floor and delivered it to the technician who measured the oxygen and carbon dioxide in the blood specimen. The whole procedure, including the usual delays encountered in finding the blood gas laboratory

66   and technician, calibrating the instrument, measuring, and waiting for the result to be printed out on a report form, took probably no more than 10 or 15 minutes, but during that time the patient died. "I rushed back to the patient's room, but my team wasn't there. The patient and his bed were not even there! And I had this blood gas report in my hand, but I didn't know what to do with it."

On another occasion, a medical student returned to his hospital ward after a weekend off, only to find that one of his patients had died. He said softly, "If only they had stopped for a minute during rounds to say something, it would have been better."

These brief incidents stand out in my memory as the starting point of an awareness of the way in which doctors and nurses in hospitals respond to death by "moving on," not leaving room or time to sort out their emotions. It seems to me that many of us find we are "holding a blood gas report" and don't know what to do with it. I carried these stories for several years before I recognized a way in which I had come to feel more comfortable with some of the emotional issues related to the death of patients. This recognition was sparked by a story told by one of our interns. It was early in the year, she was still inexperienced and unsure of herself. She had taken care of an elderly man for several weeks as he grew more ill. It was not a surprise when he died late one evening, long after his family had gone home. "My resident told me to telephone the family to tell them the bad news. I knew that this was something I should be able to do, but I didn't feel ready. I had spoken with the patient's wife only once or twice, and I didn't feel that I really knew her . . . or her husband. I was nervous as I made the call, heard the phone ringing, and recognized the wife's voice at the other end. As I began to stumble through my prepared message, I heard her gasp and cut me off saying, 'I know, he's dead.' She hung up, and I was left sitting there holding the phone. I was very angry that my resident had left it to me to make such a call."

The anger and pain on her face were fresh and evident to all in the room. The death of her patient had been expected, but the intern admitted she was "not really prepared." Having to be the "bearer of bad news" is very hard, but even more upsetting for her was the abrupt way in which the phone call ended. Why was this phone call so painful for her? As the group fell silent, I sat, mentally running my memory "in rapid reverse" to identify a like experience or emotional response that would help me to identify with and understand her discomfort and pain. I suddenly realized that something I had learned or, more correctly, had stumbled onto early in my internship had helped me to deal with the death of some of my patients.

During the 1960s, when I was a house officer, it was considered very important to perform an autopsy when any patient died. Medicine has relied heavily on autopsies to elucidate details of puzzling clinical cases, and for centuries progress in medical science was deeply indebted to families for permission to examine tissues obtained at postmortem examinations. Though modern diagnostic tools and biochemical and immunologic techniques today can provide much of the same information, autopsies still contribute to the advancement of knowledge in medicine. The difficult task of obtaining consent from a family member to perform an autopsy usually fell to the intern or resident. In preparation for requesting this consent I always met with the family and entered into some discussion about the patient's life before the illness and how he or she had coped with the illness. It often seemed that the family or friends wanted to paint a fuller picture of the patient, whom I came to know only near the end of life. These meetings added a dimension to my understanding of the patient who had been under my care. During the brief span of ten or twenty minutes there was time for reminiscence, acknowledgment, and expressions of gratitude. I know well that not all memories are sweet and not all dying is painless and peaceful, but I confess that I cannot recall any of these discussions that focused on anger or recrimination. This process of meeting the family and sharing stories about the patient, in preparation for asking consent to perform an autopsy, served as a means of dealing with my own, and possibly the families', feelings of loss in much the same ways as a *shiva* visit, the traditional Jewish condolence call.[1] Interestingly, as I reflect on this, I had come to appreciate the value of these meetings with families well before I became aware of what I believe to be the profound psychological and emotional value of shiva.

68   But dealing with death is at most a single frame of the more extended process of dealing with dying. It is the only opportunity to have a final condolence visit with families, and today's students and house staff miss it completely. But this is the last of the missed opportunities. Today's house staff often do not have the chance to develop a relationship with their patient's family while the patient is dying. In large part this is a consequence of the nature of hospital practice today with its focus, paradoxically, on both intensive care and pressure for shorter length of stay. Medical intensive care units, which are the site of many (or most?) hospital deaths, may contribute to the failure of physicians and families to arrive at common understandings of and preparation for death. The new class of "intensivists" and nurses who staff ICUs find a fundamental contradiction in preparing for death while practicing "intensive care." Patients in intensive care units are often under the care of multiple subspecialists, a circumstance that lends itself to each specialist focusing on a single organ system or problem, leaving little role for the physician "taking care of the *patient*." Visiting in ICUs is usually limited to short periods, each hour or two, and families are generally requested to leave the bedside when it appears that the patient is about to die. In the intensive care unit, death is viewed, by physicians, nurses, and family or friends alike, as a "defeat," however hopeless the prognosis and inevitable the outcome might have been. Physicians who have had a long relationship with the patient will usually find some way to communicate with the patient's family or friends to achieve some form of closure. Unfortunately, medical students, house staff, and the nurses working in intensive care units are often "left holding the blood gas report."

The Narrative Instinct

When you ask a healthy person how they feel, the answer is usually simple, "fine" or perhaps even "terrific," but if that person is ill, the response, more often than not, will be a story, a reason why they are not well, a narrative.

The writings of Robert Coles, Kathryn Hunter, and many others speak clearly and directly about the importance of narrative for the patient and to many important roles served by narrative in the relationship between physicians and patients.[1] Howard Brody wrote, "The story of diagnosis must mesh with the story of illness in a way that is more than metaphorical. It might be argued that storytelling is such a broad term . . . that there is no place in medicine where one could *not* be said to be telling stories of one sort or another."[2]

Bruner termed narrative "one of the most powerful discourse forms in human communication."[3] Narrative is a form of storytelling with origins in the earliest records of human societies. Storytelling and narrative in writings such as the Gilgamesh, the Hebrew Bible and the commentaries that comprise the Talmud, the Iliad and the Odyssey serve the

70   important function of teaching and instructing. Some teachings, such as the Ten Commandments, are presented as a list and some as simple declarative statements, but these appear to be the exceptions to the near-universal role served by narrative and storytelling as a way of teaching in all documented human cultures.[4]

Why should this be? The very universality of narrative suggests that it might have a structural basis in the human brain. Conceptual models which seek to explain mental processes often combine features drawn from what is known about information transfer in other biological systems and details taken from the way computers are programmed to process information. In recent years, we have learned much about the way information is transferred from one type of cell to another within the immune system.[5] The "information" derived from each foreign antigen must be presented to the lymphocyte in a very specific form in order to trigger the immune response.[6] If narrative serves the function of information transfer, it may be that the structural basis for its universality will be found in a specific part of the language area or another region of the cerebral cortex configured or somehow "organized" to accept and process data or input only when it is presented in some "narrative-like" form in the same way as a T lymphocyte is programmed to accept information presented in a defined form. Noam Chomsky, in explaining the acquisition of language by young children, postulated the existence of a "grammar module," an area of the brain that functions in a way that allows syntactic patterns to be distilled from speech and generalized to facilitate the acquisition of language.[7] Steven Pinker expanded this concept and suggested the existence of other "mental modules" that might serve different information processing tasks.[8] Pinker did not postulate a "narrative module" but this seems a likely candidate to consider. Taking the model of the brain as a "super parallel computer," the universality of narrative might be attributed to a "hard-wired program" designed to run software programs (learning) only when the information is presented in a specific format (narrative).

The reader, at this point, may choose to reject both the concept of "mental modules" and the tenuous analogy between the brain and a

computer with hard-wired circuits. Just as the universal distinction between "up" and "down" is almost certainly a consequence of the fact that
we are all subject to the same laws of gravity, the universality of narrative
may simply reflect the universal conditioning of infants and children who
are instructed early in life by stories, fables, and fairy tales. Jerome Bruner
described narrative as one of "certain classes of meaning to which human
beings are innately tuned" in a way that precedes the acquisition of
language.[9]

However one conceives of the basis for universality, there can be little
question that narrative serves an important role in human communication, teaching, and learning, and nowhere is this truer than in the narrative of a patient's illness. For this reason, it troubles me to realize that the
patient narrative in medicine has much in common with the ozone layer
and the tropical rain forest. Although their importance is clearly evident,
each seems to be greatly threatened by the forces of "progress." What
threatens storytelling and narrative? Physicians have always known that
imbedded within the patient's narrative are words and phrases that direct
the listener to the general or even the very specific medical problems of
the patient. Interviewing a patient requires the physician to pay close
attention to a unique detailed sequence of events while interweaving a
series of directed questions that lead from the imbedded clues to the formulation and exploration of a differential diagnosis. As medicine comes
to understand disease processes, there is a tendency to substitute that
understanding for the unique, unpredictable, uncanny sequence of events
that make up the narrative, the experience of illness. In psychology, the
analogy drawn between thought processes and computer logic has led to
the idea that the brain truly functions as a computer and that phenomena
that cannot readily be computed—meaning, values—are seen as epiphe-
nomena or illusory.

The central role of narrative in medicine is threatened by the reductionism that inevitably, and perhaps appropriately, follows the identification of fundamental unifying cellular and molecular mechanisms. It is
also threatened by the advent of technologies that make it simple to
"unlock clinical data from narrative reports."[10] Computer programs are

72   being developed that can extract information from natural language. The word-processing program I use (evidence that I am not a total Luddite) allows me to check spelling and could easily be expanded to identify words or phrases I have used in excess or incorrectly, as judged by a programmed set of grammar rules. Natural language processors armed with a glossary of technical terms and a few rules of grammar and syntax, though still rudimentary, electronically scan the dictated reports of radiologists, pathologists, or other physicians and extract specific information from the narrative.[11] The application of such computer technology to natural language makes it a simple matter to generate diagnostic codes for billing purposes or to retrieve data for statistical analysis. The possible applications of natural language processing, boggle the mind. Many of these applications will be very valuable, others may be more problematic. It troubles me to think that natural language processing will come to be used to "unlock clinical data" from the patient's narrative. This seems inevitable; it will be heralded, by some, as "efficient," "objective," "unbiased," and "reproducible." However, those parts of the narrative that will be left behind, probably to be discarded after the key words or phrases have been picked out, are rich and valuable for both the patient and the physician, and they should not be lost.[12]

As a teacher, I am equally concerned that the narrative, an important mode of instruction, will be replaced by algorithms and decision trees. *If a decision tree falls in the forest, does it make a choice?* Natural language processors will be able to generate lists by scanning everything from textbooks to the Gilgamesh. Natural language processing could probably generate a list of the Ten Commandments from the Bible and, as programs improve, might also come out with lists of the animals that should not be eaten and sexual relations that should be avoided. Replacing narrative with lists and tables is attractive in that it seems to put the world at one's fingertips. However, if there is a mental "narrative module" or an innate readiness to process information presented as narrative, we could be in for a lot of trouble.

Imagine a "future medicine" in which patients enter their stories into a natural language processor that "unlocks" the narrative to generate a list of differential diagnoses complete with mathematical probabilities, computer-generated pertinent literature references, an evidence-based algorithm for treatment and a running total of the time consumed by the "medical encounter." But my sense is that the narrative instinct, whatever its basis, is strong and not easily suppressed. People everywhere seem to be telling or writing stories.

My recent experiences in a course devoted to teaching patient interviewing tell me that the instinct for narrative is as strong as ever for patients and physicians. A faculty of almost fifty physicians, drawn from medicine, pediatrics, surgery, obstetrics, neurology, psychiatry and anesthesiology, spanning a spectrum from senior full professors to two gifted second-year fellows met almost weekly during the first three months of the school year to interview patients with groups of three or four first-year medical students. For the first session with my group, I introduced Liz, Annie, and Jason to a man in his late thirties, who had recently received a cadaveric renal transplant. I explained that they were medical students, early in their first year, interested in hearing about his illness. He began by asking whether any of them knew anything about lupus. When this was met by silence, he proceeded with a short medical explanation, "It's a disease in which your immune system reacts against your body. In my case it caused a lot of trouble with my kidneys." He went on to describe how, when he was a teenager, he developed lupus with renal involvement. His disease was severe and virtually unrelenting. He required treatment with large doses of medications (corticosteroids), which caused his bones to become soft and necessitated the use of a cane. "I was pretty weak and I could not get around well enough to go to school, so a teacher had to come to our home every day. It was pretty rough in those days. When my older brothers and sister came home from school and went out to play, that's when my teacher would come. I actually could not go out in the sun anyway . . . that's another thing about lupus. The hardest thing was when they began to go out on dates. I thought that was something that would never happen to me . . . but actually I did eventually meet someone and I was really lucky. She was willing to marry me even though it looked as if I was going to need dialysis for my kidneys.

74   When it happened, dialysis wasn't too bad. I was able to keep working [at a bank]. My doctor, who had seen me through all those years finally agreed that I should try a kidney transplant. I was on the waiting list for a kidney, but I began to have trouble with blood clots in the arm they used for my dialysis—they said it was a problem connected to my lupus. During the summer I was in the hospital almost every other week for an operation to open a clotted blood vessel. They told me it was going to take two years to get a kidney. I knew I would never live that long the way things were going. I went home one day and wrote to the head of the transplant program and explained my problem. I asked if there was anything that could be done for me, because I was not going to make it. The next week I got this call to come in—they had a kidney for me."

The students stood motionless and completely absorbed, their initial uneasiness no longer evident, as they listened to his story. I knew the patient's history and had spoken with him before this student interview session, but I was equally moved by what I was hearing. He went on to describe some of the misgivings he felt about petitioning for special consideration, but then he proudly announced, "I am making urine again, and I had not done that in more than a year." I could not tell whether the students were going to cry or cheer. Before we left they asked a few questions about how it felt to be a patient from such an early age, and the patient asked them about their initial responses to medical school. I sat with the students outside the patient's room to review what we had heard. This was our first session, and they were a bit hesitant. They seemed overwhelmed by what they had heard. Slowly they identified important themes in the patient's powerful narrative. They had all sensed an excitement in the patient's voice that seemed to go beyond what they expected with the return of renal function and good health. Jason said softly, "Some people take the bull by the horns. He finally took something back from the disease which had taken so much from him."

This patient's story was like a gift. Each session I spent with the three students was rich in narrative, moving and instructive for all of us. The stories could fill a book, perhaps they will someday. The powerful effects of hearing patient narratives came through in many of the short essays that the students submitted at the end of the course. One wrote

When you listen to the older patients, you realize that they've gone through everything you are going to go through. It's like when you come out of a movie which you loved so much that you did not want it to end. You look at the people waiting in line for the next showing and envy them because they are about to have a great two hours, but its over for you. You know how it ends. You can watch it over again, but it will never be the same as the first time. That is how I think the older people we interviewed feel when they talk to young people like us. And I imagine that's how I'll feel in fifty years.

It was not only the medical students who were moved by the experience of listening closely to the stories of patients. Faculty members, most of them with many years of clinical experience, described the sense of rediscovery and exhilaration they felt in listening to these narratives with young medical students. "It was like watching a child see a butterfly for the first time," explained one of the faculty. Another said, "I learned it was important not to focus too much on specific diseases or the medical history . . . it was more important to get them to have the courage to probe patients when the going got rough, and to tune into their personal attitudes and feelings about patients' biographies, lifestyles, suffering, and denial. The quote that kept coming back to my mind throughout this course was one by Albert Schweitzer—something to the effect that 'setting a good example isn't just one way to change another person—it's the only way.'" The responses of our faculty were quite similar to the responses of physicians who served as mentors in the Harvard New Pathway program. It was noted that "many participating physicians comment that the course has revitalized their commitment to medicine and teaching."[13]

These experiences serve as a reaffirmation that the instinct for narrative is sufficiently strong that, given any opportunity, like small trees that grow in the narrow spaces between large stones on the mountainside, it will flourish and serve both patients and their doctors.

The Whole Truth . . . ?

The attitudes and expectations of patients and physicians with regard to revealing the truth have undergone dramatic changes over the past twenty-five years. When I was a medical student, house officer, and a young physician, the prevailing dictum (or so I believed) was that the truth should be used judiciously, as with any treatment administered by the physician. Patients rarely questioned the actions of their physicians. The word *cancer* was rarely spoken and patients usually were told that radiation treatments, hormones, or chemotherapeutic drugs were given to "prevent problems." The prevailing notion today is very different. Paternalism has been rejected in favor of patient autonomy and the view that "full disclosure" is requisite for good medical practice.[1] Greatly increased patient awareness of sophisticated issues regarding diagnostic and treatment aspects of many illnesses is in part responsible for the dramatic change in the role of truth in the physician–patient relationship. In no small degree this shift can also be traced to the climate of fear of malpractice actions in medicine today.

I was totally unprepared when Mr. N's wife said bluntly to me, "You cannot tell him that he has cancer." Mr. N, a Hungarian-born lawyer in his seventies, had been under my care for about ten years. He had mild high blood pressure but had been generally well and was still working at his law practice. He had noted a persistent cough and fever for several weeks. A chest X-ray revealed a small patch of pneumonia. When he failed to improve with antibiotic treatment he was hospitalized; a CT scan of the chest revealed several masses in his lungs. After some hesitation, he agreed to a transthoracic needle biopsy. He was still in the hospital when the pathology report indicating "well-differentiated adenocarcinoma" returned. Mr. N's wife, whom I had met many times during his office visits over the years, was waiting for me outside her husband's room. I explained that the lung biopsy had confirmed my suspicion of a malignancy. She asked what I intended to do, and I explained that there were further diagnostic tests that should be performed. She was attentive but showed little emotional response until she stated, in a manner which made it quite clear that she was well prepared for this moment, that under no circumstances was I to tell her husband the diagnosis. She stated that he would not question my ordering further X-rays or other tests (looking for a primary lesion) if I explained that they were "necessary for further treatment." I tried to convince her that it was important for me to maintain an honest relationship with Mr. N. I explained that although no further treatment was required at this time, my deception would be apparent as his disease progressed and would then make it difficult for me to care for him. She had obviously prepared herself for this argument too and said, simply, that she would worry about that in the future and would find, perhaps with my help, another physician at such time. I said I would delay for a while my discussion with her husband, and we agreed to talk, in my office, the following day. Long discussions with my wife and with one of my colleagues with a strong background in bioethics did not make the matter much clearer for me. When we met the following day, Mrs. N explained that her husband had always been given to periods of depression; she feared that hearing that he had cancer might "push him over the edge." This judgment was confirmed by a phone call to Mr. N's daughter and to a physician who had treated him for depression some years earlier. Still, I wondered if Mrs. N was acting in her husband's best interest or in her own. Was she simply

78   denying the terrible fact that he had metastatic cancer and, in a way, forcing me to be an accomplice in that denial? Although Mrs. N. had always seemed a bit impatient with and critical of her husband, as we went on it became clear to me that she was in fact intensely devoted to her husband and was committed to protecting him at any cost. The repercussions when the deception was revealed would surely be worse for her than for me. Yet I found myself struggling to find some way to convince Mrs. N that her husband should be told that he had cancer. Reluctantly I agreed to a course of action that would have been my first response twenty years earlier, but now left me unsure and uncomfortable. I have often thought back on my decision. I presented the problem at several of our Humanistic Medicine seminars. All agreed that it was clearly a "difficult situation." No clear ethical guidelines seemed to emerge.

Mr. N accepted the news that he had a "complicated pneumonia" and that, after completing a course of antibiotics, he could leave the hospital to be followed in my office. The next year was uneventful for Mr. N; he came to see me for regular visits every two or three months and never again commented about his "pneumonia." About eighteen months later, Mrs. N called to report that her husband was admitted to another hospital, critically ill with anemia and jaundice. He died several days later. Mrs. N thanked me for the care I had given to her husband. Something in her tone of voice or language, I thought, also expressed her gratitude for agreeing to withhold the diagnosis from her husband. I recognize, in retrospect, that Mrs. N was probably correct in her judgment, and I came to respect the strength with which she resisted the arguments I had presented in a manner that was intended to imply that they reflected the best opinion of the medical community. Was it reasonable for me to decide, unilaterally, that he should be told the truth in order to protect the integrity of my relationship with him? My long discussions with Mrs. N made it clear that although Mr. N was my patient and his wife was not, they had shared a long, rich, and, at times, difficult life together. In the end I think it was the realization that I had a responsibility to Mrs. N, as well as to my patient, that governed my decision.

The issue of truth telling in medicine is not simple. Today most physicians would argue that patients should be fully informed. Paternalism, despite its linguistic roots in the word *pater* (father), has become anathema. The potential risks or side effects of every treatment, no matter how unlikely, are usually described in considerable detail before obtaining the patient's consent. When such warnings are affixed to cigarette packs or bottles of alcohol, the intent is to discourage smoking and to dissuade pregnant women from consuming alcohol. However, when the patient with intractable angina is advised that coronary angiography or angioplasty may lead to an arterial embolus, to the loss of a limb, or might necessitate emergency coronary bypass surgery, the intent behind presenting this catalogue of potential catastrophes is not to discourage the patient from undergoing the procedure. Nor can it can be honestly claimed that the recitation of this litany of possible disastrous complications is intended to give the patient the opportunity to make an "informed judgment." Although this information is always presented in the guise of full disclosure and truth telling, the underlying motive has more to do with "documentation." Patients are not allowed to choose whether they wish to hear all of the potential hazards of the procedure they are about to undergo! It has been suggested that this "truth telling" and informed consent be witnessed by a third party or even videotaped! The motive behind this routine practice is not simple, but truth telling and full disclosure are the norm in relations between patients and physicians today and in my view reflect a serious breakdown in this relationship.

I find that I do not feel the same need to detail all the potential complications of a procedure or treatment that I have advised for my patient as do the consulting invasive cardiologist or the consulting oncologist. I can hear my reader murmuring, critically, "paternalism." Reflecting on my own life and the medical encounters of members of my family, I am not sure that I am ready to reject a measure of paternalism. Our society cannot and should not return to the time, not very long ago, when patients were told very little and were expected to listen to the advice of a physician "who knew best."[2] I do, however, think something important has been lost when a physician feels that every doubt and concern, however remote, unlikely, or frightening, must be shared with

80   the patient. This form of presenting the "whole truth" to the patient bears a striking resemblance to the manner in which the *Physicians' Desk Reference (PDR)* lists all the potential side effects of each drug. While it may be appropriate for the *PDR* (and I have some doubts even about this!), I surely do not feel that the physician should "reveal all" just as a package insert does. "Truth" and "facts" are not discrete, defined entities, like so many colored marbles, to be handed to the patient to accept or reject. The words physicians speak to patients often linger in their minds and in their memories. They are repeated, examined, and reexamined, as patients seek reassurance, guidance, or solace. We have all heard our own words or the words of other physicians repeated by patients, years after they were spoken. I am quite sure that there are times when what has been said has had greater consequences for the patient's well-being than the medications or treatments prescribed. It seems to me that what is said to a patient or a patient's family should reflect the physician's fullest understanding of the patient's needs in the same way that the choice of a medication or advice regarding surgery does. For some patients this will require "full disclosure," by which I mean an effort to fully educate the patient, recalling that the linguistic root of the word *doctor* is *docere,* meaning "to teach." For other patients, or under other circumstances, it may be more appropriate to use the truth judiciously. The decision is not a simple one and, I submit, cannot be made according to a uniform rule or universal principle. The issue has been made much more difficult by the fact that less than full disclosure has been judged, at times, as malpractice. The decisions of how much truth is called for or is appropriate, like the question of how much treatment is appropriate, should reflect the physician's fullest understanding of the patient's life rather than society's current attitudes about paternalism and truth telling.

AIDS

I feel nothing but revulsion toward AIDS, a disease that in this country per-
versely culls the young, the vivid, the joies of our vivre. AIDS has throttled hope
and baffled medical science, destroying the brief illusion that the age of infectious diseases was behind us. Nor has the tragedy brought us together and
inspired us to new heights of generosity, insight and empathy. If anything,
AIDS has strengthened old partitions between people and constructed a few
of its own: between straights and gays, between the poor and the well-to-do.
Natalie Angier, The Beauty of the Beastly

AIDS made its appearance in New York in 1981. From the outset,
Bellevue Hospital and New York University Medical Center have been
at the very center of the epidemic. The impact of AIDS on its victims and
on the health care system has been devastating, but the effects of the epidemic on medical students and physicians have been equally profound.

At the orientation meeting for each group of third-year students beginning their clerkship on the medical wards, we carefully review a series of safety precautions. "Gloves must be worn, needles should not be   81

82   recapped, all used needles must be placed in designated containers for disposal, students who are uncomfortable drawing blood from any patient should request that the subintern (a fourth-year student), intern, or resident perform the venipuncture." These are all sensible precautions which reduce the risk of exposure to HIV-infected blood. Medical students, house staff, nurses, and other hospital personnel know that only rarely does HIV infection follow a needle stick; nevertheless, the specter of the inadvertent needle stick is pervasive. The concern among my medical school classmates was tuberculosis. My tuberculin skin test turned positive at the end of my third-year clerkships; this was not at all unusual. We were observed, but not treated. I recall that some of our teachers, addressing our fears of contracting tuberculosis, would remind us that several of their classmates and colleagues credited a year spent in a TB sanatorium with having provided them with the opportunity to delve into a subject that changed the course of their lives. The fear of contracting AIDS cannot be romanticized or glorified in this manner. At this time AIDS is incurable and fatal and any "change in the course of life" that follows HIV infection will almost certainly be a disastrous one.

The fears associated with drawing blood from patients who are known to be, or even suspected to be, infected with HIV cannot be understood solely in terms of the statistical likelihood of a needle stick or the probability that a needle stick will result in infection. It seems rather that the fear arises from some deeper sense of directly confronting the full terrifying picture of AIDS and the blood that bears the terrible offending virus. The safety precautions—gloves, double gloving, needle guards, face masks, and plastic visors employed in hospitals—are not sufficient to give a real sense of safety when drawing blood from a patient with AIDS. To feel "safe" from AIDS requires more than physical barriers. Different, more complex, coping mechanisms are needed for young physicians who witness a steady parade of young patients with a disease that, before their eyes, causes such profound suffering and physical deterioration. Anxiety about the possibility of acquiring HIV infection through a needle stick seems to evoke a strong, healthy measure of denial. Several published studies based on questionnaires suggest that interns and residents generally underestimate the risk of acquiring HIV infection through a needle stick but demonstrate a great deal of concern about acquiring AIDS.[1] Students and house officers draw clear distinctions between "them" (the patients) and "us" (the doctors). They stress the connection between HIV infection and "lifestyles." Patients who use illicit drugs, regardless of whether they are known to have used intravenous drugs, are called "IVDA's" (intravenous drug abusers). The problem of drawing the line between "them" and "us" becomes more difficult when the HIV infection has been sexually transmitted. Medical students and physicians are uncomfortable asking patients about their sexual behavior or preferences. For some the suspicion that the patient might be homosexual or promiscuous (however defined) or might engage in "unsafe sex" (however defined) serves as a reassuring barrier between "them" and "us" or "me." The narratives of patients who seem to have acquired HIV infection as a result of heterosexual relations are met with a mixture of doubt and suspicion.

But drawing a sharp distinction between the patient and the doctor is not unique to caring for patients with AIDS. It is seen in many commonly accepted hospital procedures: patients wear pajamas or gowns, doctors wear white coats (or scrub suits); patients wear their names on wrist bands, physicians have name tags on their coats; and so on. Some distinctions between physician and patient are useful in that they serve to reduce the discomfort connected with physical and emotional intimacy and protect the sensibilities of both the patient and the physician. Some distinctions, like the physical barriers provided by latex gloves, face masks, and visors, make us feel safe from the terrifying illnesses and suffering that we witness. On the other hand, terms such as IVDA, "shooter," and "street person," which are often applied to patients with AIDS and which may provide the student or physician with a protective shell, serve at the same time, as an outlet for frustration or anger, diminishing and dehumanizing the patient. But while these responses may seem to provide some immediate defense or barrier, they leave the physician feeling diminished and less worthy. If, as I strongly suspect, the relationship with the patient is an important source of emotional sustenance

84 for physicians, this self-protective distancing deprives them of a rich source of gratification in their work.

For a medical school faculty to address only the mechanical safety measures necessary to avoid exposure to HIV infection, while failing to deal with the pervasive fear of the disease is to confront only part of the problem. To deal with the fear of HIV involves facing the existential fear of one's own mortality. Rather than epidemiologists, infectious disease experts, and oncologists perhaps philosophers or even patients themselves should instruct our students and their mentors. Over the past few years, I have come to recognize that some gravely ill patients arrive at a kind of understanding which, though largely unspoken or unarticulated, reveals great courage. Faced with real uncertainty and doubt, they mobilize their own strengths, draw support from those around them and become resolute. It is not easy to identify the sources of such courage. Facing death from illness is much the same as facing death on the battlefield. It makes heroes of some men and women. We should listen to their narratives and seek to understand the motivations and strategies of such heroes of the war with illness, just as we value the stories of our military heroes. Their strengths help them to cope somehow with unimaginable suffering. Their strengths also make it easier for us to care for them, reminding us that our role goes beyond diagnosis, treatment, and cure.

The lessons learned from exceptionally courageous patients are, I believe, very important in the education of the physician. In caring for such undaunted patients, physicians at times experience a visceral, emotional response, a deep wordless communication that is warm and sustaining. These emotional "connexions"[2] serve to replenish valuable emotional energy for both patient and physician.

A Marriage Without Divorce

Mrs. M was severely uremic with nausea, itching, and generalized edema when I met her. Born in Vienna some eighty years earlier, she had been the wife of a Russian artist until his death twenty years earlier and was herself formerly a fabric designer. A fiercely independent woman, she lived alone and had no family, but several younger friends were devoted to her. She was very ill and worn out by the ceaseless itching and the difficulty she experienced moving between the second floor walk-up apartment in which she lived and the small studio where her late husband's paintings still hung. She listened as I explained that she would need dialysis treatment. With little enthusiasm, but with a brief flash of the sharp wit I came to recognize as part of her very rich and cultured life, she observed that "dialysis is a marriage without divorce." At the time I took the remark as the first step in her acceptance of this treatment which, I explained, would not be simple but would probably make her feel considerably better.

From my perspective over the next three years, hemodialysis and the associated treatments, including vitamin D, calcium, iron, and erythro-

86 poietin, did much to relieve Mrs. M. of the worst symptoms of uremia, but her course was not uneventful. Hospitalizations on several occasions—for cardiac arrhythmias, chest pain, and vitamin D intoxication—gave me many opportunities to watch her muster her strength and recover after brief periods when it appeared that the end was in sight. At times she appeared to be an isolated, utterly confused, frail old woman. Before my eyes in the hospital, for reasons which I could not always identify, she would rally and once again become a very knowledgeable artist, eager to educate me concerning the unique qualities of Matisse's collages and anxious to hear about my two granddaughters.

Mrs. M. is one of those patients with whom physicians develop a special relationship. I recognize that, as a physician, I have often been encouraged by her favorable responses to treatment, even though it was not clear that her improvement was attributable to my good care. It has been more difficult to accept my patient's own less rosy assessment of her health. At such times, on arriving at my office and after commenting on the "interesting" combination of shirt and necktie I am wearing or inquiring about my family, she looks at me sadly to ask, "Will it ever be better than it is now?" My response, generally, is to list the many features of her uremic state that have responded to dialysis, "You no longer have intense itching; you were covered with scratch marks. You are no longer swollen or breathless. You have gained weight and seem stronger," and on it goes. As I finish my list of things which are better, she turns to me with a knowing look and simply states, "But there is little that I am able to do; where will it end?" When she first asked this question, I had no answer; nor could I respond the next several times. After much thought, I decided earlier this year to reply to her question, not as though it was an existential cry but rather as the serious inquiry of a woman who had lived a long, rich, and at times difficult life. I recalled for her that she had once characterized dialysis, as "a marriage without divorce." Taking a deep breath, fearful that I was about to take a step that might lead to unexpected places, I stated, "There is always the option of divorce: you could choose to stop dialysis treatment." This was not meant to be a challenge to her, a threat that she might die if she rejected my treatment. I intended to begin

a discussion of the options, and Mrs. M, sensing this, asked, "How long
would it be, I mean how long could I live without dialysis?" My response
was guarded, "Weeks, possibly months." "Will it be very unpleasant . . .
the dying?" I assured her that I would continue to treat her and would do
everything in my power to keep her comfortable. I think I detected a
twinkle in her eye as she responded, "I don't think I'm ready for divorce
yet." This "contract" has been reviewed, and the terms reaffirmed once
or twice during the past year. I do not believe that Mrs. M. feels any
better, but I sense that the understanding we reached made living a little
easier.

Shaky Evidence

When I first heard the term *evidence-based medicine,* it barely caused a ripple in my consciousness. There is nothing novel in the idea that decisions should be based on evidence. But the longer I pondered the concept, the more I realized that something did not sit just right. If evidence-based medicine was a new paradigm, what was it intended to replace? The lead article in a major medical journal announced, "A new paradigm for medical practice is emerging. Evidence-based medicine de-emphasizes intuition, unsystematic clinical experience, and pathophysiologic rationale as sufficient grounds for clinical decision making and stresses the examination of evidence from clinical research."[1] As described by the Evidence-Based Medicine Working Group, the term is somewhat of a misnomer since it focuses, almost completely, on a narrow, albeit important, aspect of medicine, namely clinical decision making. It ignores the much larger role of medicine as a discipline that seeks to expand the scientific understanding of human disease and to develop new, more effective therapies. It seems a far cry from the care of patients in a relationship in which the physician must seek to attain what Sherwin Nuland

88

described as a "a sensitivity to medical decision-making that transcends   89
the mere clinical facts of a patient's illness and conscious motivation that
would seem to determine choice of treatment options."[2]

As outlined by the Working Group, the major features that form the
basis for evidence-based medicine consist of greater reliance on published
clinical trials and attention to critical analysis of these studies using basic
principles collectively termed "clinical epidemiology." A cursory review
of the monthly contents of major medical journals or a casual cruise along
the information highway via MEDLINE, will convince any reader that
the medical literature is increasingly dominated by reports of large, multi-
center, randomized treatment trials and retrospective analyses of large
data sets. Computer-assisted access to the findings of randomized treatment trials, together with improved methodologies to analyze the data
from such studies, facilitate interpreting the findings and appropriately
applying the conclusions to clinical decision making. Together, these
comprise the centerpiece of the new paradigm.

What is wrong with the paradigm of evidence-based medicine? First,
clinical trials are of very limited value in clinical decision making. The
very design of such studies makes it impossible to apply the findings to
most patients. Patients enrolled in most clinical trials have been selected
because they do not have any of a long list of coexisting or comorbid
conditions that could possibly confound the interpretation of the findings
or might make adverse responses more likely. Unfortunately, patients
often have these troublesome comorbid conditions. The hallmark of a
well-designed clinical trial is that it asks a very narrowly defined question
that can be answered by the data. The number of variables examined is,
by design, kept to a minimum. For many patients, by contrast, these
unmeasured or unexamined variables may be of greater importance in
determining outcome. Often the measured end point is only a surrogate
for an important end point that cannot be readily determined or that
might require a much longer treatment trial. Although this form of study
design often yields unequivocal answers to defined questions, these are
not what we need when we look for help in choosing a therapy for a
single patient. Many of the clinical questions where "evidence" would be

90 most helpful cannot be answered from clinical trials because controlled studies have not or cannot be carried out for ethical or practical reasons.

In recent years, when the data available from clinical trials has been inconclusive, statisticians have resorted to the technique of meta-analysis.[3] This statistical approach is based on the (unlikely) assumption that a data analyst can pool the findings of many small inconclusive studies to yield a large, unbiased body of data from which statistically significant conclusions may be drawn. But, since the data that is pooled, that is, the data from smaller published studies, has already been subjected to selection by reviewers and editors of other journals, bias cannot be avoided.

Even more troubling when we seek to base decisions on the findings of published clinical trials is the fact that today many of the large multi-center, randomized clinical treatment trials are designed, financed and guided, either directly or indirectly, by the pharmaceutical industry which, by establishing the trial design, may bias the "evidence." Physicians and patients alike recognize the limitations of large clinical trials in clinical decision making. This is readily seen in the ongoing debate, in both the medical literature and the lay press, concerning important issues such as the use of hormone replacement therapy in postmenopausal women or the effects of dietary antioxidants in cancer prevention.

Enough about statistics, statisticians, and treatment trials. The statement that the new paradigm of evidence-based medicine is intended to free decision making from its dependence on "intuition, unsystematic clinical experience, and pathophysiologic rationale" is even more disturbing. "Intuition and unsystematic clinical experience" often represent the keen observations of a single observer rather than the recorded findings of an army of health-care providers checking off boxes on questionnaires and forms. These unique observations have already been pushed to a marginal position by the Biomolecular Revolution and the introduction into medicine of many powerful new diagnostic modalities. Are these time-proven aspects of medical care to be challenged now by a paradigm that is fundamentally opposed to the growth of science and technology in medicine? The paradigm that evidence-based medicine is intended to supplant is a tradition of medicine based on the implicit assumption that progress in the treatment of disease comes from greater understanding of the pathophysiology of the disease. It is a tradition that rests on the careful observations and intuitions of great clinicians such as Charcot, Osler, and Cushing and of countless lesser-known physicians who, in the past and today, have been serious students of medicine. Their "unsystematic observations" have been pursued in the laboratory by clinician-scientists and basic scientists—physiologists, immunologists, biochemists, pharmacologists, and, more recently, by geneticists and cellular and molecular biologists. The result has been the gradual evolution of Western medicine which, though still limited by vast areas of ignorance, has as its central core a growing body of scientific knowledge of the pathophysiology of disease. We are still very far from a full understanding, and therefore rational therapy, for most chronic diseases. At times this has led physicians, acting independently or in droves, to advocate therapies that seem arbitrary, irrational, or downright useless. The alternative approach, that is, to systematize our ignorance and elevate the limited findings of randomized clinical trials to the level of guiding principles, strikes me as a great mistake, one that gives a new meaning to the descriptive term "double blind."

My concerns about the challenge that evidence-based medicine poses go much deeper, however. In the preface to *Acts of Meaning* Jerome Bruner wrote, "Books are like mountaintops jutting out of the sea. Self-contained islands though they may seem, they are upthrusts of an underlying geography that is at once local and, for all that, a part of a universal pattern . . . they are part of a more general intellectual geography."[4] I would paraphrase Bruner's statement to read, "Ideas and new paradigms are like mountaintops." I see the call to evidence-based medicine as part of a larger "underlying geography," a geography whose landscape extends well beyond the issue of clinical decision making. The same arguments that have been marshalled in support of evidence-based medicine are repeated in the growing arena of "outcomes-research."[5] Outcomes-research aims to derive algorithms and guidelines for patient care from data obtained by reviewing the medical records of Medicare patients or other large patient groups. Webster's dictionary defines the term *data* as

92   "things known, from which inferences may be deduced." In science data is assumed to be collected by careful observation or measurement, hopefully free of observer bias. The data, culled from patient records and coded by individuals whose training is not standardized, whose performance may or may not be closely supervised, is not likely to be free of bias since the diagnostic coding provides the basis for physician and hospital reimbursement. This data has been used to assess the appropriateness of specific forms of medical or surgical treatment and to compare the quality of care given by different physicians, in different hospitals, and in different areas of the country. The statisticians responsible for this sort of data analysis give their assurance that the outcome measures are "adjusted" for differences in the severity and complexity of illness encountered in different practices, hospitals, and geographic regions. The validity of such statistical "adjustments" is clearly open to question,[6] and I have the distinct impression that these results are viewed with distrust by all but the inner circles of statisticians who generate this type of data. If it is possible to "adjust" for all these variables, why do other statisticians need to go to such lengths to design randomized double-blind trials that assure comparable control and experimental groups? Despite these limitations, outcomes-research data constitute the basis from which guidelines for the treatment of specific diseases are now being formulated. These guidelines, which generally also incorporate considerations of cost, choice of drugs, length of hospital stay, and inpatient or outpatient setting for procedures, have been seized upon (if not actually generated) by government health care financing agencies and for-profit health care organizations.[7] It does not require a great leap of imagination to see that these guidelines will easily be translated into algorithms for care and will finally be promulgated as components of medical education. Algorithm-driven medical care and algorithm-driven medical education are ideas that might have had their origins in the imagination of George Orwell.

    Evidence-based medicine and outcomes-research have already created an adversarial climate in medicine. While it is obvious to all that consensus guidelines do not represent either "the truth" or even a unanimous viewpoint, these guidelines impose standards and patterns of care that are unacceptable for many patients and physicians. Patients often find legal means to press for insurance coverage for forms of therapy that the consensus guidelines deem "experimental," for example, intensive chemotherapy and autologous bone marrow transplantation for some malignancies. Physicians with recognized expertise in specific areas may take public issue with consensus guidelines. Some argue their position in the media and others in medical journals. Others can only grumble. As a medical student, I heard a story told of one of my teachers who was asked, during his certification examination in internal medicine, whether he would give digitalis or quinidine for a specific condition. When he answered "digitalis," the examiner criticized him stating, "Paul Dudley White (a highly respected leader in cardiology at the time) would give quinidine." My teacher, a crusty man even when he was young, fired back, "Let him!" Readiness to question expert opinion is always healthy in medicine. But it is a far cry from the assertion that experts should be rejected as "authorities" and the claim that evidence-based medicine aims to replace "authoritarian medicine" with "authoritative medicine."[8] I find this a serious and frightening claim. Equating expertise with authoritarianism, and the findings of randomized multicenter trials with authority, carries very strong overtones of anti-intellectualism.

The rejection of expertise as "authority" connects, in my mind, with a larger segment of Bruner's "underlying geography," namely with the growing movement of irrationalism and antiscientific thinking that was the subject of a recent three-day meeting at the New York Academy of Science.[9] The geography, as I perceive it, stretches from distrust of expertise in medicine and the promotion of a wide range of "alternative therapies" to the emergence of postmodern science, the notion that all science is "subjective" since humans cannot perceive the world directly. It seems a cruel irony that this antiscientific movement should surface and gain prominence at a time when advances in the biologic sciences make it virtually certain that we will soon understand normal function and disease at a much more fundamental level and have effective treatments for diseases for which we must now make do with randomized treatment trials and alternative medicine.

94   I think things will come out all right, and it will be precisely because of the new science and technology. Medicine at this time is expensive and frustrating. There are more treatments and more diseases that can be treated, but few cures. Coronary bypass surgery, renal dialysis, organ transplantation, joint replacement, cancer chemotherapy, and vasodilator therapy for the treatment of congestive heart failure are all remarkable advances in medical therapy, but the cost is great and none actually cure the underlying disease. If it were not for the introduction of the polio vaccine, which effectively eliminated paralytic poliomyelitis, the treatment today would consist of lifelong respirator therapy for most patients with respiratory paralysis, more radical experimental attempts to implant diaphragmatic pacemakers for a few, and many forms of "alternative medicine." I suspect that we would be hearing a great deal about the cost to society, priorities, and the need for cooperative clinical trials and consensus guidelines to determine which of these "halfway technologies" to recommend.[10] Fortunately Salk and Sabin pursued their visions of a vaccine. The development of truly curative treatments, which will inevitably come as a consequence of the remarkable recent events in genetics, cell and molecular biology, is exactly what is needed to transform the "underlying geography" of medicine and society.

A Critical Incident

More than thirty years have passed since I was an intern, but a brief incident on the oncology ward is so vivid in my mind that I can still feel my skin tingle when I recall it. The chief of service, Dr. Daniel Laszlo, was making his weekly rounds with a retinue of fellows and house staff. A much respected and revered man, Dr. Laszlo had done important clinical research on cancer and enjoyed a reputation as both a great clinician and a scientist. As the group moved from bed to bed in the large ward, Dr. Laszlo listened to brief summaries of each patient's problem, progress, and treatment plan. It was not only the medical staff that stood close by to catch every word or question spoken by "the chief." There was a general hush over the ward as other patients and nurses seemed to respond to the moment as well. As the group began to move on to the next bed, Dr. Laszlo paused and returned to the elderly woman with metastatic breast cancer that had become unresponsive to hormonal therapy. He leaned close to hear her softly spoken words. He gently removed her dentures and placed them in a cup on her bedside table. She smiled as he rejoined the large group making rounds.

96   I often remember this brief episode, not so much for the sensitivity and kindness shown by "the chief," but because I feel that such a gesture by the chief of service commands special attention. To this day I marvel at and envy Dr. Laszlo's ability to "hear the soft voice in a noisy room." I often thought about what special qualities were required to have this unique sensitivity. I stumbled upon a partial answer, quite by accident, when I recalled one of my earliest experiences, as a medical student learning physical diagnosis. For a beginner in medicine, each portion of the physical examination was very detailed, and it seemed that, unless parts of the examination were omitted or done in a less than thorough manner, a full physical examination would require many hours. A highly respected cardiologist spent an hour with my small physical diagnosis group demonstrating the examination of the heart. He pointed out that the murmur of mitral stenosis was, at times, difficult to hear because it was confined to a very small area. "The murmur might be hidden under a quarter," he said. One of us, probably not me, had the temerity to ask how one could ever find it if it required such a meticulous search over the patient's chest. He pointedly stated, "You search when you suspect it will be found." Some years later these words connected in my mind with the incident on the oncology ward. Dr. Laszlo was a fine, sensitive physician, but he was also highly skilled and experienced in the treatment of patients with terminal cancer. He knew when to expect that poor nutrition and chemotherapy might leave a patient with painful oral ulcers. He could hear the soft voice in the same way that the professor of cardiology could hear the low pitched rumble of mitral stenosis on a noisy medical ward. The seemingly small gestures and occasional very sharp observations are important because they are evidence, both to me as a physician and to my patients, of medicine being practiced in a way that engages my fullest emotional and intellectual capacities. These moments are in the nature of epiphanies. They create lasting memories and can change the lives of physicians, patients, and students.

     I will never know whether Dr. Laszlo was aware of the effect his action might have had on the minds and future behavior of some of his colleagues and students. Just as memories of the incident have resonated in my behavior with patients, the incident has led me to ask what I might do that could so touch and change students and young physicians with whom I come in contact. In medicine, both the development of awareness and sensitivity to the needs of patients and the understanding of underlying disease processes seem to progress in a slow, almost imperceptible, fashion punctuated by rare and dramatic transforming "breakthroughs." The formulation of the germ theory, the identification of hormone receptors and second messengers, and the revelation of the genetic code transformed science and medicine. In the development of the physician, the "breakthroughs" are individual epiphanies. A student observes a respected professor in a special moment and is changed as permanently as the scientific world was changed by the report of Watson and Crick. How is it possible, as a teacher, to create such moments? It seems to me that the same kind of preparation and willingness to engage one's intellect and emotion in patient care that I recognized in watching Dr. Laszlo may be the necessary first ingredients in teaching. Epiphanies don't occur with great regularity, but they are transforming experiences for those who are fortunate enough to experience them. Perhaps this is a clue as to why medical students seem to learn so much more from patients and from their mentors than from the best organized textbooks, lectures, or computer programs.

The Homeless Man on Morning Rounds

Where is there a story that paints a true picture that is not worth reading?

Samuel Lowenstein, "My Early Life" (unpublished)

Morning rounds, after a day when six or seven new patients have been admitted, are invariably busy. There is much work to be done, tests to be requested, consults to be arranged. Over the years, the house staff have developed ways of streamlining the presentation of the new patients on attending rounds in order to avoid "getting bogged down in details." All extraneous information is omitted. Interns, or medical students if they are chosen to present a new patient, are carefully instructed to present the patient's history, physical finding, and laboratory values in a style that appears to lead, like a highway, directly to the diagnosis—with no detours. For several years, I've been aware of this shared understanding, and, in a way, I have benefited from this efficient style, since it kept my morning rounds at Bellevue from running over into the mid-afternoon.

I hadn't really planned it, but as the intern began presenting "a middle-aged homeless black man," I asked what she meant by "homeless." "Un-domiciled" she responded, then reading my facial expression, she slowed down and explained that he had been living on the street. She knew that he had come to New York within the past few months, that he had no home and had lived in parks and on the street. Where did he live before that? I could feel her searching back into the memory of her interview with the patient, the previous day. She recalled that he had come from California and, yes, that he had something to do with making films. My interest was aroused, but I had to wait as the intern resumed her presentation of his initial complaints ("cough and fever") and the other details of his history, physical findings, blood test results, and chest X-ray. When we, a group which included two residents, two interns, and two fourth-year students, went to the patient's bed, I asked how long he had been in New York. I admit to a certain curiosity about people who are "un-domiciled," but I am uncomfortable asking, in front of others, where a person lives when they are "on the street." The patient replied that he had been "here for a few months." His next response, that he had come from California was similarly matter-of-fact. He seemed to become more engaged with our group when asked what he did in California. His answer that he had "made some films" led me to ask, hesitantly, what sort of films and whether I might have seen one. He mentioned a very successful movie. He had us now! "Do you remember, it was with——?[1] There was a scene where this fellah comes up and talks with her in a bar, well, that was me." Some wished that we could pursue this much further, but I went "back to business," listened to his chest, and we moved on to the next patient to be presented.

Did that small exchange add measurably to the diagnosis? I suppose one could find a way to bring together this man's history as an actor who played a small part in a film with the illness that brought him to Bellevue, but the point of the story is different. Several days later, the same intern announced on morning rounds, that she had rented the video of the film on her free evening. "It was true, there was Mr. J, just as he said, asking her to dance with him"! Our patient went on to have a long and difficult hospital course. I think that the brief exchange at his bedside had a significant effect on the doctors who took care of him. The intern saw

100 him as an individual, and that recognition translated into care that was more compassionate and attentive to the needs of Mr. J and more gratifying, albeit as it evolved, more painful for the intern.

The message seems so obvious that the telling of it makes me uncomfortable. We all know that the fears, anxiety, and loneliness of patients are greatly heightened by feelings of anonymity. Every patient has a name and a story, yet many seem to remain almost as nameless as patients who are brought in, comatose, to the emergency room as "unknown white female." Is it simply that "there is so much to be done" or that "it is necessary to be very efficient" in the care of patients? These are explanations that I often hear. I recall how one of our residents explained it. She said that as she began to interview a patient, she recognized that the patient had much to say. "If I had let her tell me her story, I would have been there all evening, and I still had four more patients to admit."

It is hard to argue with this explanation. I have wondered at times how I would respond if, one morning, the intern or resident informed me that there had not been enough time to thoroughly examine the last two patients admitted to the service because the patient he or she was caring for took so much time and attention. Would I understand, and would it matter to me whether the patient who needed "so much time and attention" was suffering from deep terror or grief which called for human contact, comfort, and reassurance or diabetic ketoacidosis which called for close monitoring of insulin therapy and fluid and electrolyte replacement? I don't know how I would respond. We all feel that every patient admitted to the hospital should be seen and attended to promptly, but we recognize that some emergencies must take precedence. Few will die of terror or grief, but patients do die of ketoacidosis, you say. Diabetic ketoacidosis is serious and life-threatening and can be effectively treated. I am troubled by the realization that these responses betray the lower priority which I, and my colleagues, accord to the clear and important role of the physician in providing comfort and reassurance to patients experiencing terror or grief. But I have presented this as an all-or-none, either-or choice. In reality I do not believe that the choices we make or the priorities we set most of the time are so black and white, whether they involve responding to the terror or to the severe metabolic acidosis. The priorities we must establish are not exclusive but rather they dictate what comes first, what takes precedence. While I have heard the complaint that there "was no time to set priorities," I have found that for me it is quite the other way around. The busier and more hectic my life, the more critical it is that I be able to establish priorities. Some would call it "maintaining control." Where in this list of priorities do I see the value of establishing "the identity" of my patient and how much importance do I place on responding to the terror I hear? The answer in part depends on the competing priorities, but if listening to the patient and being there when the patient needs comfort are to be anywhere on the list of priorities, they must first be in the mind of the physician. The challenge to the skill and sensitivity of the physician is not to choose but rather to respond, as much as possible, to the needs of the patient. This may include, under some circumstances, making it clear that the patient's needs have been deferred but not ignored. Sometimes others, physicians, nurses, friends, or family can be recruited to help.

Though morning rounds at Bellevue are still demanding and require that much be accomplished in a limited time, I think the homeless man seen on morning rounds taught some of us an important lesson, which made those rounds richer and more valuable.

Numbers, Numbers

It is hard to avoid the conclusion that our culture has become increasingly obsessed with numbers. Computers seem to be everywhere these days—home computers, laptop computers, wristwatch computers, computers on wagons in food markets. These remarkably useful devices generate numbers, quantitative information that has come to occupy an increasingly important place in our thinking. Exercise is gauged by the increase in heart rate or "mets" attained rather than the feelings of exhilaration, fatigue, or exhaustion. In medicine the increasing dependence on technology and quantitation is evident in the near-obsession many physicians and patients have with small differences in blood pressure or levels of "good" and "bad" cholesterol. I use the term *obsession* to emphasize that although differences in blood pressure of only 5 mm Hg or in LDL cholesterol of only 5 mg/deciliter are of clear-cut prognostic significance in studies of large populations, changes in blood pressure or cholesterol of such small magnitude have far less meaning for an individual patient. The concern with quantitative information and technology has resulted in the expectation, on the part of *both* physicians and patients, that medical care must necessarily rely on close monitoring of changes in blood chemistry, blood pressure, and the like and requires us to depend heavily on these diagnostic tools. Patients, too, have become "obsessed" with quantitative data. In a scenario that is only a little exaggerated, the patient, when asked, "How are you?" answers, "You tell me," and the physician, after reviewing the results of a battery of blood tests, responds reassuringly, "You are fine." You will argue that the greater availability and use of routine blood testing has led to earlier detection of diseases. "Suppose that the day comes when these diagnostic tests are widely available, accurate, easily affordable, and are accomplished rapidly and safely. Would that not be progress?" I think not. The tacit assumption that "quantitative data" is somehow better or more important than qualitative or "narrative" information is wrong and misleading. Teaching on the medical wards, I have found this to be dramatically illustrated in the way students and house staff typically assess a patient who presents with the complaint of chest pain. The feature that is stressed is usually the intensity of chest pressure or pain, which is typically described as "8 of 10" (severe), or "2 of 10" (mild). There is a double fallacy in this, now almost universal, "quantitative" approach. First, it assumes that the severity of chest pain is closely correlated with the likelihood that the pain is of cardiac rather than noncardiac origin. This is simply wrong. Further, it should be obvious that the pain may be graded as "2" by one person and as "8" by another, because each person is comparing the discomfort with their own prior experience. It is not that quantitative assessments by patients are unimportant or unreliable but that these measures only have value in the context of the individual patient's narrative. Pain experienced in different settings might be rated as "8" or "2" by the same patient. Chest pain, which awakens an elderly person living alone during the night is very likely to be rated as more severe than pain the following day when the sun is shining and a family member is present. Using these "pseudoquantitative" descriptions as objective measures not only wastes time and intellectual effort but leads to erroneous conclusions. The "number" given to the patient's chest pain often overshadows some of the other terms which describe the quality of the pain—what it felt like—which are

104 usually more helpful in ascertaining the cause of the symptom. The practice of describing chest pain in numerical terms has become so pervasive that patients who have had repeated visits to the Emergency Room often come in complaining of "8 out of 10 chest pain."

The consequences of our obsession with numbers go beyond the tendency to replace vivid, revealing qualitative description with sterile numbers. Although I recognize the value in using an abridged or shorthand account when time is limited, I am concerned that quantitative information is judged as more important, reliable, or valid than qualitative or narrative data in arriving at decisions in medicine. A close friend who is an excellent, thoughtful cardiologist confirmed this impression for me. He acknowledged that in deciding whether a patient was suffering from digoxin toxicity, the finding of an elevated blood level of digoxin in an asymptomatic patient would be much more likely to lead him to change therapy than would the typical symptoms of digoxin toxicity in a patient whose plasma concentration of digoxin fell within the accepted therapeutic range. More detailed quantitative information, including some measure of receptor number, affinity and occupancy by digoxin, and possibly some measure of the activity of the enzyme system (sodium-potassium ATPase), which is inhibited by digoxin, would yield a very precise measure of the effects or toxicity of digoxin, but the limited information given by the plasma concentration of the drug alone leads to a false sense of understanding and, at times, to incorrect therapeutic decisions.

But, it might be argued, pursuing the example of digoxin toxicity, when technology is sufficiently refined and when tissue or receptor concentrations of drugs can be measured, "science" (read "numbers" or quantitative data) and not "art" (read the patient's narrative) will be the best way to ascertain whether the dose of digoxin should be changed. If this is taken to mean that given enough "hard science," molecular and cell biology, the patient's narrative will be less important in medical care, I must strongly disagree. While the precise measurement of a series of biochemical and membrane changes may fully define a complex biological phenomenon, such as that which follows the complete cessation of blood flow to a portion of the heart muscle, and while these "numbers" relate this event to all other like events in the heart, the experience of a heart attack is unique for the patient. New diagnostic tests and a deeper understanding of physiologic processes greatly enhance our ability to diagnose accurately and to treat effectively, but they cannot fully address the unique aspects of illness that bring the patient and the physician into a relationship whose importance is not diminished as medicine becomes more "scientific."

As difficult as it may be to create or to maintain such hybrid creatures, it is critical that physicians caring for patients in this era of the Biomedical Revolution be able to fully understand "the numbers" while retaining their sensitivity to the unique aspects of illness.

Alternative Medicine

I was both bemused and shocked when I learned that the National Institutes of Health had created an office of alternative medicine. The idea of "alternative" medicine leaves me feeling ambivalent and angry. Widely discussed in the media, increasingly the subject of editorials, news releases, and clinical studies in medical journals, the term *alternative medicine* encompasses a wide range of concepts in health care and a myriad of treatment modalities including relaxation therapy, chiropractic, acupuncture, t'ai chi, homeopathy, biofeedback, bioelectromagnetics, guided imagery, and therapeutic touch. What features justify lumping or grouping these diverse concepts and therapies under the unifying term *alternative medicine*? The history of Western medicine has been one of a continuing series of "alternative" intellectual constructs and forms of treatment. Phlebotomy, leeches, and purging were replaced by more effective alternative therapies. The germ theory, the recognition of the role of the immune system, and the pioneering studies that led to the correlation of specific areas of the brain with specific neurologic defects or seizure disorders all represented forms of "alternative medicine." Because they were found to be more effective or were more concordant with broader beliefs within the medical scientific community, they superseded earlier medical beliefs and practices. This has not always been an imperceptible gradual evolution. Some alternative therapies emerge over a short time to challenge and replace existing traditional treatments. Clearly the term *alternative medicine* means something other than the evolution of new and better treatments or a new way of viewing the pathogenesis of a specific disorder.

Many of the entities subsumed under the rubric alternative medicine—such as acupuncture, moxibustion, t'ai chi, and some forms of herbal medicine—have their origins in Eastern or Chinese traditional medicine. By "origins" I mean that the understanding of the underlying diseases, their pathogenesis and manifestations, and the appropriate therapies are closely linked to a much wider, pervasive view of the organization of the body and its functions. As clearly as the ancient Greek concept of humors dominated the thinking and treatments of physicians in the time of Hippocrates, the concepts of "chi" or Yin and Yang are the pervasive determinants in the classification and therapeutic approach to illness (and wellness) in traditional Chinese medicine. Is this what is meant by alternative medicine? I do not believe that most advocates of "alternative medicine" are merely voicing their preference for Eastern medicine over "the narrow chauvinistic approach of Western medicine with its emphasis on the scientific method."

Some would find it more correct to characterize alternative medicine as a system of thought and treatments based on constructs that place greater emphasis on the relation between the mind and the body. There is little doubt that Western philosophy has long been dominated by mind-body dualism and that this underlies many of the paradigms by which we understand disease and its treatments. Admittedly, even as I write these words, I find it difficult to fully equate the processes of formulating my thoughts and putting the words on paper as simply two comparable sets of biomolecular events, cellular interactions, and organ activities. But although burdened by the intellectual legacy of mind-body dualism embodied in, "I think therefore I am" rather than "I am, therefore I am,"

108   traditional Western medicine has been able to make significant progress in understanding the physical basis of thoughts, emotions, and memory. Long before advocates of alternative medicine began to call for greater attention to the interaction of mind and body or to denounce mind-body dualism, conventional medicine was pursuing a course of investigation that, in its early days identified the basis for psychosomatic disorders in the altered activity of the autonomic nervous system and identified gross anatomic lesions in the brain as the cause for specific behavioral changes. This tradition of investigation has led in recent years to a recognition of the unique localization of "mental processes" in specific areas of the intact brain, to the beginnings of a notion of how learning and memory are represented by molecular transformations in synaptic clefts, and to the identification of chemical transmitters, common to "the mind" and "the body" that are responsible for cell-to cell communication.

Those who champion "mind-body medicine" as the alternative to traditional Western medicine focus on the failure of "organized" medicine to recognize the importance of factors related to the physician-patient interaction, relaxation, stress, mental attitudes, and social support systems in the overall response of patients to illness and to treatment. I strongly suspect that these variables play a considerable role in both the pathogenesis and the outcome of a great many diseases. However, neither the scientific findings, for example, that lymphocytes have adrenergic receptors or that the number of natural killer cells may be subject to behavioral modification, nor the clinical studies that demonstrate the beneficial effects of support groups on the survival or level of performance of patients with cancer seem sufficient grounds to establish a new "alternative" category of medical treatment. I think the same arguments could be used to reject the identification of holistic medicine as a medical system that claims to take more of the patient into consideration as alternative medicine.

It seems to me, rather, that alternative medicine is a rallying point, an entity created to serve as an umbrella or, better yet, a magnet that brings together many very different forms of alternative treatments. Rather than a common therapeutic concept, the commonalities among these different entities may be found in their rejection of some, most, or all of traditional, or as it is more often expressed, "organized" medicine. I do not intend to reject, in a sweeping generalization, all of alternative medicine. If attention to micronutrients, biomagnetism, or positive imagery are believed to be important in the treatment of patients, advocates or champions for these modalities must convince open-minded people of the efficacy or value of these therapies or new treatments if any of them is to become widely accepted. Leaders in the alternative medicine movement point out that the clear benefit of many generally accepted forms of treatment—psychoanalysis, cardiovascular fitness exercises, or vitamin supplements—has never been established by rigorous clinical trials. Further, they assert correctly that the efficacy of some modalities of treatment, such as acupuncture or biofeedback, are not easily tested in traditional double-blind, placebo-controlled trials. This represents a challenge to those who believe that their alternative therapies have beneficial effects. Objective evidence must be adduced if any of these modalities is to be generally accepted. The lack of rigorous scientific evidence of the clinical efficacy for accepted forms of treatment (psychoanalysis, fitness exercises, or vitamin therapy) has, in fact, kept them from being universally accepted by the public, by physicians, and by the insurance companies that pay the bills for health care. To designate a treatment as alternative medicine does not allow one to bypass this requirement, nor does the conviction based on one's philosophical belief system that such therapies hold some promise justify declaring the existence of a new entity, alternative medicine. How then do we account for the growing network of advocates of different forms of therapy, the establishment of courses in alternative medicine as part of medical school curricula, a Center for Mind-Body Medicine, and an office of Alternative Medicine at the National Institutes of Health? Seen in its best light, the answer might be that this represents a groundswell of committed individuals coming together with a common purpose. I do not believe this is the case. I see the growth of alternative medicine as the development of a

110   network whose goals are related to issues of power and money along with individual ego and ambition, the same forces that are evident in traditional medicine.

The alternative medicine network generates further support and creates the appearance of substantiality. Major foundations have, for a variety of reasons, lent support to the alternative medicine movement. A cadre of leaders in the nascent field can already be identified. Some of these emerging leaders may have a uniquely far-reaching understanding of illness and will ultimately be credited with significant contributions to the progress of medicine. Even if this proves to be true, I cannot accept the validity of the designation alternative medicine or its watered-down equivalent, "complementary medicine." The notion that alternative medicine is the way to address the care of chronic illness and the failures of society to cope with issues of loss, isolation, and progressive disability, and to claim that this "alternative" form of care is more cost-effective and humane than medicine as it is generally practiced,[1] even if it were true, which it is not, creates a disruptive and destructive dichotomy. It is this deepest resonance and undertone of the term *alternative* that troubles me most. I welcome any new insights or understanding that lead physicians to be more sensitive and patient care to be more effective, more compassionate, more holistic, or more affordable but I reject the view that this is alternative medicine—it is simply progress in good medical care.

Bellevue Hospital

Bellevue Hospital has been the epicenter of my life in medicine for forty years. One hears a great deal these days about how changes in health care delivery will affect the training of house staff and the impact of changes in health care financing on large urban hospitals. Not all of the news is good, and some is very worrisome. Whatever changes come about in these next few years, Bellevue, the major teaching hospital of New York University Medical Center, will remain for many of us a vast, exciting, frightening, challenging world-unto-itself.

A true picture of Bellevue Hospital cannot be constructed from the statistics—the number of admissions, the ethnic diversity of its patient population, or even the sociology of this hospital which has cared in turn for each successive immigrant group that has come to the United States, settled in New York, and learned to find Bellevue Hospital when they became ill. My picture of Bellevue is a quilt-like composite of recalled incidents and images. I suppose an anthropologist might liken Bellevue Hospital to a self-contained society, unique in that it is not off in some remote area of the world but is set smack in the middle of a busy modern

112   city. From my perspective such a sociologic or anthropologic view misses the main point. Bellevue Hospital has been the training place for countless young physicians (and nurses) over the course of its rich 250-year history. While the demography of the East Side of New York City has changed and the patient population has seen, in fits and starts, both gradual evolution and radical changes, an army of young men and women have come from everywhere to spend the most formative years of their lives learning to care for patients. Medicine is not learned from textbooks. Osler wrote, "To study the phenomena of disease without books is to sail an uncharted sea, while to study books without patients is not to go to sea at all."[1] Even close contact with a diverse patient population and dedicated teachers would not train students to become excellent dedicated physicians if it did not take place within a setting in which medicine was being practiced, not simply taught. To train at Bellevue Hospital is to enter into a world which is, at once, chaotic, demanding, alienating, seductive, and exotic. Young physicians who train at Bellevue cannot help but be touched and changed, in some way, by this environment.

My earliest recollections of Bellevue Hospital, the "old hospital" that was Bellevue before the present modern building was opened in 1975, dates to my first year in school when on Saturday mornings we came from the medical school building across the street to the Bellevue Clinic building for "clinical correlation." A patient, whose disease related in some way to the subjects we were studying, was presented to us and discussed. I remember the elevator in the clinic building had two signs. One, directing patients to the medical clinics on the fourth, fifth, and sixth floors, was printed in English, Italian, Chinese, and Yiddish. Below it, a battered, hand-lettered sign read "Ring Up for Down." The patients, in the hallways and those brought to our clinic conference, looked vaguely like my grandparents and were very deferential to the doctors. One of the first patients I ever examined, as a second-year student, was on a large open ward at Bellevue Hospital. The short, gray-haired cardiologist who was my physical diagnosis instructor was his doctor in the Cardiac Clinic. Dr. Bertha Rader had cared for him for many years and was responsible for his having been admitted to Bellevue at this time for heart surgery, the repair of a rheumatic valve. He was very patient and somewhat bemused as six medical students in turn struggled to hear and then identify his heart murmur. The unspoken, but evident, understanding between this burly retired policeman and our physical diagnosis instructor made it quite clear that teaching, learning, and patient care were being combined seamlessly. This observation, which seems as natural to me as the changing tides for one who lives at the edge of the ocean, may require some explanation for the next generation of students and teachers if medicine comes to be an elaborately choreographed dance of health care providers and consumers and standardized patients. For the record, the patient trusted his cardiologist/physical diagnosis instructor; she had earned his trust and respect by her careful attention and dedicated care over many years. She remembered him clearly when I asked her as we walked together up First Avenue last month.

The two years spent as a clinical clerk on the various wards of Bellevue Hospital are dominated in my memories by an image that, unfortunately or perhaps fortunately, is a thing of the past. The wards were large rooms, accommodating from 20 to 30 beds, arranged along the side walls and down the center aisles. The nurse's desk and medication cabinets stood just within the entrance. Medical students, usually six or eight in a group, arrived each morning carrying our black bags awaiting morning rounds. Nursing students, all young women in those days, seemed equally nervous and uncomfortable as they were given assignments by their instructors. Nurses, doctors, medical and nursing students, and patients were all in plain view of each other; privacy consisted of a small screen that could be positioned around the bed of a patient being examined, undergoing a procedure, or dying. For all the indignities of being on an open ward, there were some good things about the arrangement. I do not believe patients saw a "teaching hospital," with medical students, interns, and residents responsible for their care, as a threatening place. The frequent "rounds" by house staff and medical students early each morning and later with visiting attending physicians, gave clear evidence to the patients that their care was supervised by older "gray-haired" doctors and that teaching was going on all the time. As a student I felt I was always being

114   watched. Patients often kept an eye on us, as well as on other patients who might need help.

My mind moves ahead to my years as a medical resident. The large wards were the same, but my role and responsibilities had changed dramatically. Bellevue always seemed to be busy. It never closed its doors. Patients were admitted at all hours of the night and day and, if directed to the medical services, were assigned to the next ward in rotation. You could tell the season by the length of the row of beds in the center aisle of the ward. In the winter, "pneumonia season," beds overflowed into the hallway. The challenge for a resident, even in those days before "length of stay" and DRGs (diagnosis-related groups) entered the medical lexicon, was to keep one's ward census down so the hall would not be lined with beds nor would patients need to be "boarded" on other floors of the hospital. Some of us were very good at managing the flow of patients, others, and I was one, found this difficult, as I still do. It seems that almost everyone who has ever trained at Bellevue has stories to tell. For me, after the unforgettable incidents and the patients, many of whose names linger in my mind, I am left with memories of comradery, midnight meals, and the realization that during the three years spent as a medical resident learning medicine, I began to experience the unique satisfaction of teaching. My role models always seemed to excel in the dual roles of physician and teacher. I recall standing, for what seemed like hours, with Dr. William Goldring, a very crusty, demanding senior physician, trying to give a coherent explanation of the significance of a patient's distended jugular veins. He challenged every statement and made me examine the logic of each assumption. I can still see his gnarled fingers and wry smile as he taught the fundamentals of cardiac hemodynamics in heart failure at a patient's bedside. Nor can I forget rounds with Dr. Alfred Vogl, another great teacher and outstanding physician. I had presented, with excitement, the history and findings of a young woman, an alcoholic, who came to the hospital with recurrent venous thrombosis. We suspected an underlying malignancy. Having heard the details of her case, Dr. Vogl entered the patient's room, looked at the pale, disheveled woman with her alabaster complexion and uncombed, bleached blond hair, and said softly, "She looks as though she stepped out of a Botticelli painting." It seemed to come out of the blue, but I knew what he meant. There was no special clue to the diagnosis to be found in the woman's appearance, but Dr. Vogl saw her, not with the tunnel vision of a medical specialist, but with the full power of observation that reflected his rich intellect. Sometimes this makes all the difference, and in that moment I learned something about looking at a patient that has remained with me to the present.

As a senior resident, making rounds with a man who in today's parlance might be termed a "world-class cardiologist," I described hearing a heart murmur. When Dr. Kossman listened and disagreed, I backed off saying I was probably wrong. He smiled, cautioned me not to give up so easily and explained that "even the last place baseball team beats the league leader two or three times each season." Without seeing myself as "the league leader," I have frequently recalled this incident on my teaching rounds with students as I encourage them to think and to challenge. When I find myself becoming overly concerned with broad issues of curriculum or the use of computers in teaching, I am brought back to the realization that lessons such as these taught by respected physicians in the setting of ward rounds or around a patient's bed were an irreplaceable part of my medical education.

As a resident I saw many patients with alcohol- and drug-related problems. The alcoholics came to the hospital with delirium tremors, seizures, pneumonia, or hypothermia; there were always a few patients with advanced cirrhosis, easily identified by their hollowed cheeks, scrawny arms and legs and a large protuberant abdomen, who "bounced back" into the hospital each time they were discharged. Drug addicts, mostly heroin users, were not a rarity. They appeared in the emergency room with infections, occasionally with the dramatic picture of drug-related respiratory depression, or they were transferred to the Bellevue prison ward from other prison facilities with drug withdrawal or neuromuscular symptoms that looked frighteningly like those of tetanus, but almost always proved to be secondary to a medication. I don't remember feeling threatened by these patients, and I clearly recall thinking, at times, that I was like Nikolai Gogol glimpsing life in "the lower depths." Drug addicts

116 were tough patients to care for. They often needed to be treated with intravenous antibiotics for long periods of time for deep infections or endocarditis. They taxed the patience of physicians, students, and nurses alike. This has not changed, and the difficulties our students and house staff experience today in treating such patients—the constant need to deal with drug-seeking behavior, to bargain with and cajole patients in order to treat them adequately—has often been the topic of hour-long discussions in our Humanistic Medicine seminars. When the group leader summed up one such session with the observation, "You seem to have such trouble dealing, as you must, with such difficult patients—they make very great demands on your energy and your patience—and yet, it strikes me that these are the experiences you seem to enjoy the most and get the most from!" The smiles of the students were a clear acknowledgment that she was right. An important part of "the Bellevue Experience" has always been the very great involvement and effort that young physicians expend in the care of patients who are desperately ill, demanding, and difficult.

Over the years Bellevue's population has changed. There are still those older patients who remind me of my grandparents, but changes in demography, health insurance, homelessness, drug addiction, and AIDS have made Bellevue a more difficult, frightening place. Armed police are always present outside the Emergency Room and the sight of a police guard sitting outside the room of a patient on the medical or surgical service is not at all unusual. Rooms specially designed to circulate filtered air at a high flow rate for patients with drug-resistant tuberculosis and the ubiquitous red plastic containers for needles and syringes are silent reminders that we live in an environment in which it is not only the patients who are at risk. And yet it seems to me that Bellevue, in its role as a place where patient care, teaching, and learning blend, is perhaps more unique than ever. The streamlining of medical care and the increasing dependence on outpatient diagnostic facilities, day surgery, and subspecialization were not designed to facilitate medical education. Quite the contrary, medical students, interns, and residents require a slower pace or a less efficient system; their development requires daily direct patient responsibility. Bellevue, as an urban municipal hospital, still plays the role of the primary physician for most of its patients. But the patients, more than ever before, are isolated, alienated, homeless, or angry. Others are recent arrivals from China, Taiwan, Thailand, Cambodia, Vietnam, Bangladesh, Pakistan, Russia, and African countries whose names we barely recognize. Bellevue finds translators for their many languages, creating a virtual tower of Babel on First Avenue, but it remains for the students, doctors, nurses, and social workers to find a way to understand their customs, their needs, and their fears. I don't believe it is possible to care for a patient whose home is "on the street" or a patient whose home was on the Thai-Cambodian border without knowing more about the patient and where he or she lived. The lesson that caring and learning are closely linked is sometimes forgotten when there is so much to be done in a busy municipal hospital, but for me it will always be as much a part of Bellevue Hospital as the sign posted on the main elevator which read "Ring Up for Down."

Afterword

As I was completing these series of essays, a remarkable story was unfolding at Bellevue Hospital. It seemed like the completion of a circle, a perfect coda. With thoughts of the "midnight meal" and recapturing "human connexions" echoing in my mind, I read a short piece by Michael T. Kaufman in the About New York column of the *New York Times* of October 29, 1994.

Mr. Kaufman explained how David Margolis, an immigrant from Odessa who had worked as a W.P.A. artist almost sixty years ago, had painted a series of murals in the entrance rotunda of Bellevue Hospital. The artist described the painting, "I was here weekends and nights. I was painting in a place of distress. . . . So many people, so much drama. Crying, screaming, and also laughing. And in the middle I was painting murals that told the story of human progress."

The murals were lost, painted over, and covered with grease in 1945 as Bellevue Hospital was reshaped to meet the need for additional space. Earlier this year, Mr. Margolis, now eighty-three years old, began restoring the murals, just as the once stately entrance to Bellevue is being

120   restored. As Mr. Kaufman notes, "Something more than just art was being rejuvenated." And Mr. Margolis's description is perfect: "It is like finding that what you thought was dead is alive. . . . It is like finding lost friends."

    Each time I enter Bellevue Hospital and pause to look at the murals, I find myself thinking of these words, of patients who looked like my grandparents, of "human connexions," and of "midnight meals."

Notes

The Biomolecular Revolution

1. E. O. Wilson, *Naturalist* (Washington, D.C.: Island Press, 1994).
2. J. O. Watson and F. H. C. Crick, "A Structure for Deoxyribose Nucleic Acid," *Nature* 25 (1953):737–38.
3. L. Thomas, *The Youngest Science* (New York: Viking Press, 1983).
4. A. Flexner, *Medical Education in the United States and Canada* (New York: Carnegie Foundation for the Advancement of Teaching, 1910).
5. Thomas, *Youngest Science.*

Can You Teach Compassion?

1. The goal of the Program in Humanistic Medicine, initiated in 1979 for the medical service of New York University Medical Center, was to introduce into the clinical training a sanctioned meeting in which third- and fourth-year medical students and medical house staff would be able to explore aspects of their experiences that were not regularly addressed in teaching conferences, ward rounds, or meetings with attending physicians. The program was devel-

oped in the belief that the responses of medical students and young house staff who are confronting death, suffering, and grief should be acknowledged and addressed as part of their educational experience. Groups consisting of four to eight third-year medical students who comprise one or two ward teams at Bellevue Hospital or New York University Hospital meet weekly during the course of the ten-week clerkship in Medicine. Small groups of interns and residents participate in similar meetings during the periods when they are assigned to the Medical Intensive Care Unit and the AIDS Unit at Bellevue Hospital.

2. A. H. Shem, *House of God* (New York: Dell Publishing, 1981).
3. R. J. Lifton, *The Nazi Doctors* (New York: Basic Books, 1986).
4. H. Spiro, "What Is Empathy and Can It Be Taught?" *Annals of Internal Medicine* 116 (1992):843–46.
5. H. Khan and R. E. Randall, *Squash Rackets: The Khan Game* (Detroit, Mich.: Wayne State University Press, 1972).
6. D. A. Matthews, A. L. Suchman, and W. T. Branch, "Making 'Connexions': Enhancing the Therapeutic Potential of Patient-Clinician Relationships," *Annals of Internal Medicine* 118 (1993):973–77.

Coughs, Clouds, and Ice

1. In *Arctic Dreams,* Barry Lopez (New York: Bantam Books, 1987, pp. 187–92) mentions at least twenty words that the Inuits use to describe ice. I recognize that there is, within linguistic circles, considerable furor over what has been termed The Great Eskimo Vocabulary Hoax (G. K. Pullum, *The Great Eskimo Vocabulary Hoax and Other Irreverent Essays on the Study of Language* [Chicago: University of Chicago Press, 1991]). Laura Martin ("Eskimo Words for Snow": A Case Study in the Genesis and Decay of an Anthropological Example," *American Anthropologist* 88 [1986]:418–23) points out that in "Eskimo" languages words are characteristically built with multiple suffixes. Multiple words for "snow" are not in fact different from the many adjectives that modify the noun in English. Presumably the same could be said for Inuit terms for "ice." I do not pretend to be a scholar of either Inuit or Native American linguistics. Unlike some of the anthropologists, whose references to Eskimo snow words are criticized by Laura Martin, I have not tried to infer from words for clouds and ice anything about the link between the language and the culture of Native Americans or Inuits. I do, however, believe that the evolu-

tion of terms that describe coughs reflects significant changes in the culture of physicians.

Treating Chronic Illness

1. Willard Gaylin, "Faulty Diagnosis," *New York Times,* June 12, 1994.
2. T. Pincus and L. F. Callahan, "Formal Education as a Marker for Increased Mortality and Morbidity in Rheumatoid Arthritis," *Journal of Chronic Diseases* 38 (1985):973–84.

Patients as Teachers

1. Some of the names in this essay are fictitious. Although it is not my habit to call patients by their first names, there was a reason in each instance, and I have found it hard to refer to these three special patients in more formal terms. Everyone called Saul by his first name, Richard was a good friend before his illness, and Ellen requested that I use her first name. All of them knew me as Jerry.

Reassurance and the Warning on the Label

1. An extreme example of this self-protective strategy, which I do condemn, is called "hanging the crepe." The physician prepares the patient or family for the worst, knowing that if things go well everyone will be gratefully relieved.

Defending the Common Cold

1. P. F. Cohn, R. Gorlin, P. S. Vokonas, R. A. Williams, and M. V. Herman, "A Quantitative Clinical Index for the Diagnosis of Symptomatic Coronary-Artery Disease," *New England Journal of Medicine* 286 (1972):901–7.

Asymmetry

1. S. M. Rothman, *Living in the Shadow of Death* (New York: Basic Books, 1994), p. 7.
2. The program she directs is described with considerable insight and under-standing in C. Levine and M. Allen, "Social Interventions in the Care of

124   Human Immunodeficiency Virus (HIV)—Infected Pregnant Women, *Seminars in Perinatology* 19 (1995):323–29.

On Drawing Blood

1. More invasive forms of venipuncture, that is, femoral vein puncture or jugular vein puncture, are performed by more experienced physicians.
2. W. T. Branch, R. J. Pels, R. S. Lawrence, and R. Arky, "Becoming a Doctor: Critical-Incident Reports from Third-Year Medical Students, *New England Journal of Medicine* 329 (1993):1130–32.

The Vital Signs

1. R. Selzer, *Mortal Lessons* (New York: Simon and Schuster, 1974). Selzer presents a wonderful description of physical diagnosis performed by a Tibetan physician.

Holding the Blood Gas Report

1. Shiva is the Jewish traditional mourning period during which callers are expected to share a memory, a reflection, or an experience that brings the departed one into clearer focus. Rabbi A. M. Goodman, *A Plain Pine Box* (New York: Ktav Publishing House, 1981).

The Narrative Instinct

1. R. Coles, *The Call of Stories: Teaching and the Moral Imagination* (Boston: Houghton Mifflin, 1989); K. M. Hunter, *Doctors' Stories: The Narrative Structure of Medical Knowledge* (Princeton, N.J.: Princeton University Press, 1991).
2. H. Brody, *Stories of Sickness* (New Haven: Yale University Press, 1988), p. 13.
3. J. Bruner, *Acts of Meaning* (Cambridge: Harvard University Press, 1990), p. 77.
4. D. E. Brown, *Human Universals* (New York: McGraw-Hill, 1991).
5. A foreign substance or antigen (the raw information) is partially digested into small components (peptides or carbohydrates) and linked to specific cells (macrophages) in order to be presented to a processor (the T lymphocyte), which mediates the immune response through a host of chemical signals to other cells. The reader interested in a full exposition of the analogy between

information transfer in the immune system and the brain is referred to Gerald
Edelman's *Bright Air, Brilliant Fire: On the Matter of the Mind* (New York: Basic
Books, 1992).

6. H. M. Grey, A. Sette, and S. Buus, "How T Cells See Antigen," *Scientific American* 261 (1989):56–64.

7. N. Chomsky, *Language and Mind* (New York: Harcourt, Brace and World, 1968).

8. S. Pinker, *The Language Instinct* (New York: William Morrow, 1994).

9. Bruner, *Acts of Meaning,* p. 72.

10. G. Hripcsak, C. Friedman, P. O. Alderson, et al. "Unlocking Clinical Data from Narrative Reports: A Study of Natural Language Processing," *Annals of Internal Medicine* 122 (1995):681–88.

11. Physicians dictating reports seem to adopt the program of these word processors and speak in the phrases that the program seeks out; can thinking in machine language be far behind?

12. M. Viederman, "The Computer Age: Beware the Loss of the Narrative," *General Hospital Psychiatry* 17 (1995):157–59.

13. W. T. Branch et. al. "Teaching Medicine as a Human Experience: A Patient-Doctor Relationship Course for Faculty and First-Year Medical Students," *Annals of Internal Medicine* 114 (1991):482–89.

The Whole Truth . . . ?

1. It is instructive to realize that this was a bloodless revolution, a remarkable example of how, at times, a society can turn black into white without legislation, stormy protest, or any attempt at finding a consensus.

2. H. Brody, "The Chief of Medicine," *Hastings Center Report* 21:4 (1991):17–22.

AIDS

1. R. N. Link, A. R. Feingold, M. H. Charap, K. Freeman, and S. P. Shelov, "Concerns of Medical and Pediatric House Officers About Acquiring AIDS from Their Patients," *American Journal of Public Health* 78 (1988):455–59.

2. D. A. Matthews, A. L. Suchman, and W. T. Branch, "Making 'Connexions': Enhancing the Therapeutic Potential of Patient-Clinician Relationships," *Annals of Internal Medicine* 118 (1993):973–77.

1. "Evidence-Based Medicine," *Journal of the American Medical Association* 268 (1992):2420–25.
2. S. B. Nuland, *How We Die: Life's Final Chapter* (New York: Vintage Press, 1993).
3. S. N. Goodman, "Have You Ever Meta-Analysis You Didn't Like?" *Annals of Internal Medicine* 114 (1991):244–46.
4. J. Bruner, *Acts of Meaning* (Cambridge: Harvard University Press, 1990), p. ix.
5. S. Vibbert, *What Works: How Outcomes Research Will Change Medical Practice* (Knoxville, Tenn.: The Grand Rounds Press, 1993).
6. J. Green and N. Winterfeld, "Report Cards on Cardiac Surgeons: Assessing New York State's Approach," *New England Journal of Medicine* 332 (1995): 1229–32.
7. A. Epstein, "Performance Reports on Quality—Prototypes, Problems and Prospects," *New England Journal of Medicine* 333 (1995):57–61.
8. F. Davidoff, K. Case, and P. W. Fried, "Evidence-Based Medicine: Why All the Fuss?" *Annals of Internal Medicine* 122 (1995):727.
9. "Scientists Deplore Flight from Reason," *New York Times,* June 6, 1995.
10. L. Thomas, "The Technology of Medicine," in *Lives of a Cell* (New York: Bantam, 1974).

The Homeless Man on Morning Rounds

1. I have omitted the name of the actress to maintain a measure of patient confidentiality; the rest of the story is true.

Alternative Medicine

1. C. Halpern, "Mind vs. Medicine," *New York Times,* January 30, 1993.

Bellevue Hospital

1. W. Osler, "Books and Men," in *Aequanimitas, with other Addresses to Medical Students and Practitioners of Medicine,* 2d ed. (Philadelphia: Blakiston, 1906), p. 220.

Index